MARCHING PLAGUE

Germ Warfare and Global Public Health

Other Critical Art Ensemble Titles from Autonomedia

The Electronic Disturbance

Electronic Civil Disobedience and Other Unpopular Ideas

Flesh Machine
Cyborgs, Designer Babies, and New Eugenic Consciousness

Digital Resistance
Explorations in Tactical Media

The Molecular Invasion

Marching Plague
Germ Warfare and Global Public Health

Critical Art Ensemble

Autonomedia

State of the Arts

NYSCA

This publication is made possible in part with public funds from the New York State Council on the Arts, a state agency.

Autonomedia
POB 568 Williamsburgh Station
Brooklyn, New York 11211-0568 USA
info@autonomedia.org www.autonomedia.org

Printed in Canada

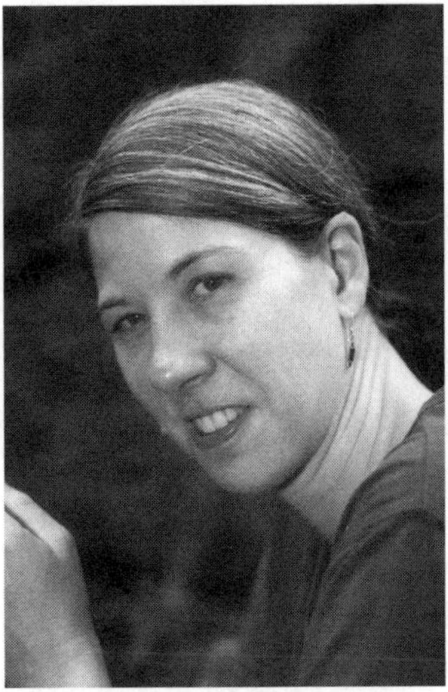

Hope Kurtz 1958–2004
R.I.P.

Acknowledgments

This book should have debuted in the late fall of 2004; instead, it makes its first showing in 2006. This late appearance, as some readers know, is due to a failed attempt by the FBI and the Department of Justice to censor this text.* During a raid on the home of Steve Kurtz, the FBI confiscated all files, notes, and books pertaining to this project. Originally, it was thought that the agency was just using these materials to make the case that Kurtz was a "political advocate" involved in terrorist plots. However, after this suspicion was shown to be little more than a paranoid fantasy, the FBI continued to hold all the materials. Consequently, CAE had to go through the unfortunate task of reconstructing the research. This process was slow, and other activities seemed continuously to get in the way—administrating the legal case, fundraising, resurrecting our projects (also lost in the FBI raid), public lectures, and wage work. CAE remained as determined as it could be under the circumstances, and *Marching Plague* is the product of this determination. The book has not turned out as we originally envisioned it, primarily because we were unable to fully reconstruct the research. In spite of all these blocks and diversions, we finally completed it to our satisfaction (albeit not 100%), along with the projects that accompany this text.

While we may pat ourselves on the back for getting this book done at all, let us assure our readers that it could never have been done without the help of so many people. Without the worldwide outcry of those who expressed outrage, sent encouragement, and created the media surrounding the case, Steve Kurtz would probably be in jail awaiting trial instead of being out in the world continuing to work with CAE. Of course, to everyone who sent money to the CAE Defense Fund to pay for his lawyers, we offer our eternal gratitude.

So many people deserve personal thanks, and none is more deserving than those who have worked tirelessly (with no end in sight) on the CAE Defense Committee. To Gregg Bordowitz, Igor Vamos, Jacques Servin, Lucia Sommer, Rich Pell, Nathan Martin, Claire Pentecost, Beatriz da Costa, Ed Cardoni, Faith Wilding, Ryan Griffis, and Greg Sholette, know that we would have been lost without you. CAE members could never have done all the work themselves. The time the defense team freed up is the time that helped make this project possible.

Thanks to NAAO, Ed Cardoni, and Polly Little for so admirably administrating the CAE Defense Fund, and keeping the IRS off our backs.

One key event contributing to creating the time to do this book was the auction/fundraiser at the Paula Cooper Gallery. For almost a year we were going month-to-month, fundraiser-to-fundraiser in order to pay the lawyer bills. This auction gave us some room to breathe. Special love to Helen Molesworth, who said an art auction could be organized to raise funds for CAE's legal defense and then made it happen. Heaps of gratitude to the auction team: Gregg Bordowitz, Sam Durant, Paula Cooper, Lucia Sommer, Doug Ashford, James Meyer, Nato Thompson, Jason Simon, Mark Dion, Ulrike Mueller, Lori Cole, Anthony Allen, Jocelyn Davis, Brooke Singer, Ed Cardoni, Wallace Shawn, the Cooper Union volunteers, and to all the artists who gave work, and all the collectors who bought it.

Many thanks to Jim Fleming and the Autonomedia collective for standing by us and publishing this book, even though it will probably mean a reactivation of the subpoena they were served. And thanks to all the people who had an impact on this book and the related projects, including Lucia Sommer, Gregg Bordowitz, Igor Vamos, Jacques Servin, Rich Pell, Nathan Martin, Claire Pentecost, Beatriz da Costa, Humberto Ramirez, Rebecca Schneider, Nato Thompson, Nicola Triscott, Rob La Frenais, Gillean Dickie, Creative Capital, Lynn Hershman, Matt Fuller, Natalie Jeremijenko, Paul Vanouse, Amanda McDonald Crowley, Stephanie Rothenberg, Adnan Hadzi, and Lennaart van Oldenborgh. We are also grateful to Jenn Phillips and Lucia Sommer who stepped in to fill the editorial void after Hope's death.

We also have to express the utmost appreciation to our longtime collaborator and co-defendant Bob Ferrell—a man whose life has been spent in the service of public health and science education, and for that, he is now an enemy of the state.

Finally, CAE must acknowledge the tragic loss of our sister in cultural arms, Hope Kurtz. She was the gateway to the public, our editor, poet, and voice of reason. Before any project was released, she reviewed all the materials, suggested necessary changes, and in the end, gave final approval. Her talent lay in her genius for pattern recognition (especially text). She could look at any kind of document, and even if she did not understand the content (which was rare), she knew if something was wrong. We called her "the voice of reason" because whenever a project was getting too abstract, specialized, or too "insiderish," she would take us to task on it. We miss her dearly and still do not know what to do without her. But even after this inconceivable loss, we continue to follow her words and vow to "never surrender" or be intimidated by the authoritarian forces that we have fought against for so long.

Critical Art Ensemble
Winter 2006

---

*For details on the illegal detention and indictment of Steve Kurtz and to support the CAE Defense Committee, visit www.caedefensefund.org.

Introduction

Bodies of Fear in a World of Threat

They wanted the Germs; they got 'em.

—Darby Crash

The use of the symbolic abstraction of fear as an exchangeable sign has always been a helpful means to justify and manifest the most perverse needs of authority invested in the expansion of militarized orders and the erasure of individual autonomy. But in the United States after the 9/11 attacks, fear reigns supreme as a fundamental unit of exchange across the entire political, economic, and military spectrum. The sign of fear filtered through the sign matrix of threat, now more than ever, not only serves the authoritarian forces of order, but the engines of profit as well. Signs such as these move at astonishing speeds through cultural and political barriers. Even the slowest bureaucracy responds to their appearance with surprising vigor, while the fastest corporate vector can use them to fuel ideological and material engines that move production and distribution at maximum velocity. Once these general signs become particularized within the narratives of body invasion and organic meltdown, opportunities for the rapid appropriation of power increase exponentially. New funds for research and the centers that house it, contracts for materials such as vaccines and symptom-arresting pharmaceuticals, security contracts, and so much more flood the marketplace to such an extent that almost every apparatus of production and service has an interest in keeping the spectacles of fear and threat in play. Whether an actual threat exists or not is irrelevant to this network of exchange. The threat of future crisis and the solution of preemptive action marches forward, gaining momentum as it goes, until it becomes a system in which so many institutions are so deeply invested that it can no longer be critically appraised. This system becomes a naturalized transparent given—a necessary fact to which all must submit lest they lose the riches that have been gained.

This is not to say that the problems and impossibilities within the system are unknown; for the most part they are, but they are not categorized as contradictions. Instead, they are presented as nonrepresentative tendencies that should be ignored. For example, one social expression of fear in a population, mass panic, has yet to be seen within the public sphere. While terrorist attacks have caused severe emotional trauma both on individual and public levels in the United States, the situation could hardly be framed as mass panic. Neither 9/11, the anthrax scare, nor the August 2003 New England blackout (at the time feared to be a terrorist action) typically has caused such behavior. In spite of (largely artificial) crises, public order has remained intact. However, those apparatuses (government, media, military, etc.) with a tremendous interest in maintaining an environment of fear encouraged the public to believe that the nonrepresentative panic buying of plastic sheets and duct tape promoted by these very institutions was proof of a grand disorder that would occur without proper vigilance and preparedness. As individuals, we suffer this contradiction between the real and the hyperreal, between spectacle and active living, in the form of a culture of waste that is grounded in the highly profitable production of the useless at the expense of the practical (better education, healthcare for all, fair wages, etc.).

Even from a military perspective, the case of germ warfare and bioterrorism is representative of the economy of uselessness. A systematic interest in this economy has oscillated between little and tremendous following the use of chemical weapons during World War I. Yet from the beginning, a constant disagreement has existed within the military as to how effective biological weapons might be. The first position taken by the United States military was that such weapons were a waste of resources. This view was best expressed by Major Leon Fox of the United States Army Medical Corps in an article written in 1932 for military surgeons entitled "Bacterial Warfare: The Use of Biological Agents in Warfare." In this article, Fox laid the foundation for what still stand as the primary arguments against the usefulness of such weapons, including the boomerang effect, bacterial sustainability, and the belief that biological weapons would not be as effective as many existing alternatives. Even at that early date, he had a degree of understanding about the production of the spectacle of fear in regard to this particular subject:

> *Bacterial warfare is one of the recent scareheads that we are being served by the pseudo-scientists who contribute to the flaming pages of the Sunday annexes syndicated over the nation's press.... I consider that it is highly questionable if biological agents are suitable for warfare.*

This position has never disappeared from United States military calculations, even during periods when germ warfare was being intensely investigated during the Cold War, after the discovery of transgenics, during the Reagan military buildup, or even today after the anthrax scare. The debate has been ongoing, yet what has sustained military efforts in this area has less to do with strategic or tactical planning and more to do with the politics of nonrational fears exchanged throughout the culture. For example, during the Cold War, research was spurred by intelligence regarding the grand scale of Soviet research and its application to weapons. This knowledge created a fear of a biological weapons gap. During this period the doctrine of preparedness (i.e., avert a future crisis by a preemptive solution) was introduced and has been in place ever since. Currently, the anthrax scare has convinced the Bush administration that even a small-scale attack could be very disruptive. The Bush administration's reaction is particularly unnerving due to the broad scope of the funding and the nature of the programs that have followed. They extend far beyond the military proper and affect public health policy.

Unfortunately, the precedent that has been set is to refuse to acknowledge this deep, long-lived contradiction of opinion over the utility of germ warfare, and this refusal is precisely what is occurring now. Nor is the artificial manufacture of fear being assessed in any way. And why would it be when there is so much profit to be made? Is it not better to go along with the situation? The public receives *ad nauseum* constant calls for preparedness as if biological attack on a massive scale is possible, as if casualty-free preparedness is possible, as if no real preparations are already in place, and as if biowarfare/ bioterrorism is a major (if not the greatest) threat to public health. Apocalypse awaits us all. For example, in their book *Germs*, Judith Miller et al. conclude:

> *If we as nation believe that the germ threat is exaggerated, we are spending too much money on it. But if the danger is real, as we [the authors] conclude it is, then the investment is too haphazard and diffuse. We remain woefully unprepared for a calamity that could make the anthrax mailings seem tame.*

The authors have made a very crafty statement. While acknowledging that other positions exist, and by seemingly taking a critical, albeit weak stand (the money isn't being spent right), in the end, they acquiesce to the apocalyptic narrative that is the foundation for what they believe to be wrong. This narrative of fear and threat is precisely the reason why the money is being misused. Threat requires action to circumvent it–not considered action, just action–for no institution that cares for the public interest can afford to be perceived as doing nothing. Of course within the context of self-interest, this narrative is also necessary to get to the top of the *New York Times* bestseller list. A call for calm is not going to be a catalyst for sales.

At other times, the agitprop surrounding germ warfare is strictly self-serving, as in this press release from the University of Pittsburgh Medical Center:

> *Bioterrorism is the greatest national security threat of the 21st Century. Bioweapons attacks could cause death and suffering on a catastrophic scale, wreak enormous economic and social disruption, and even threaten core democratic processes. Adequate response does not depend on our military strength*

but on medical and public health systems and availability of effective drugs and vaccines....

In a move that will establish the University of Pittsburgh Medical Center and the University of Pittsburgh as the international leader in the critical, high-profile, and rapidly expanding field of bioterrorism preparedness, research and response, the creation of the Center for Biosecurity of the University of Pittsburgh Medical Center was announced today.

The cynicism of such a document is nearly unspeakable. One could not ask for a greater exaggeration of a problem that has yet to exist, or a more vague implication of a means to preemptively solve it. This text is clearly guided by unrestricted self-interest masquerading as public concern.

The government is just as pleased to exploit the potential threat of germ warfare. In 1997, United States Secretary of Defense William Cohen made a dramatic appeal by appearing on television holding up a five-pound bag of sugar and declaring that this amount of anthrax sprayed from an airplane would result in the death of 50% of the population of Washington, D.C. Not only is this fear mongering irresponsible since it greatly exaggerates a highly unlikely scenario, but the information itself is incorrect. The World Heath Organization estimated that it would take 50 kilograms to cause a 20% casualty rate in a population of 500,000.

Even scientists are willing to get on board the fear-and-threat gravy train, and they will make up impossible scenarios if they have to. Consider this apocalyptic scenario from Richard Wise of the Department of Microbiology at the City Hospital in Birmingham, United Kingdom:

> *Picture the following. Over the period of about one week, increasing numbers of patients report to their general practitioners and emergency departments with fever, malaise, and myalgia, and other symptoms in keeping with viral respiratory tract infection. Increasing numbers of patients become septicaemic and then deaths start to occur. By the time the diagnosis of anthrax is made, each patient will have been in contact with many family members as well as with colleagues and people in the hospital. The initial exposure of, say several hundred people, has now spread to many tens of thousands. Panic would ensue and hospitals would be overwhelmed....*

A very frightening scenario indeed. The one problem, of course, is that there is no evidence that anthrax can be passed from one human to another human. If several hundred people were infected that is all that would be infected. And the above quote was published in the very prestigious medical journal *The Lancet* in May 1998!

It is within this environment of fear mongering, military expansion, and corrupt economic exchange that Critical Art Ensemble (CAE) felt compelled to write a critical counternarrative. In the following pages, we will attempt to sketch an outline of why bioterrorism is a failed military strategy; why it is all but useless to terrorists; how preparedness efforts have been detrimental to public health policy; what institutions benefit from biofear; and how and why this problem will not be controlled by the "diplomatic community." We certainly realize the difficulties of the task we are undertaking. Knowledge of this subject is completely fragmented. There are as many narratives as there are players in the directing of the biological industries. Given the amount of money presently on the table, no biological or political experts can be trusted, since all suffer from a conflict of interest, and therefore must be skeptically approached. Even in matters of quantity, the situation is very imprecise. For example, how can we know how much public money is being spent on biowarfare research? Black ops aside, many of the areas under this discipline are poorly defined. Bureaucrats and beancounters can play very fast and loose with what is or isn't biowarfare research. Consequently, all we can say is that the Bush administration's biowarfare initiatives are costing taxpayers billions of dollars. How many billions is nearly impossible to determine with any reliability. Hence, we are left with few alternatives to describe what is occurring. There are stacks of primary documents and a handful of historical narratives, but in the end we can only count on our material experience in everyday life to judge whether the real or the hyperreal reigns supreme in this situation.

CAE's opinion is a simple one. We believe that biowarfare "preparedness" is a euphemism for biowartech development and the militarization of the public sphere. Preparedness, as it now stands, is a madness that continues because it gets votes for politicians, audiences for media venues, profits for corporations, and funds for militarized knowledge production. If there is any real threat to our bodies and health, it is not coming from weaponized germs, but from the institutions that benefit from this weaponization.

Note: In our discussion of public health in this book, we will not address the interrelated topic of the HIV/AIDS pandemic in any detail. Not because we do not see a connection or fail to value its significance within this discourse, but because we believe that there is adequate literature on the subject by authors far more qualified to represent the situation than ourselves.

In addition, we are only addressing germ warfare proper. We are not including chemical or toxic weapons (even if derived from a germ) in this analysis.

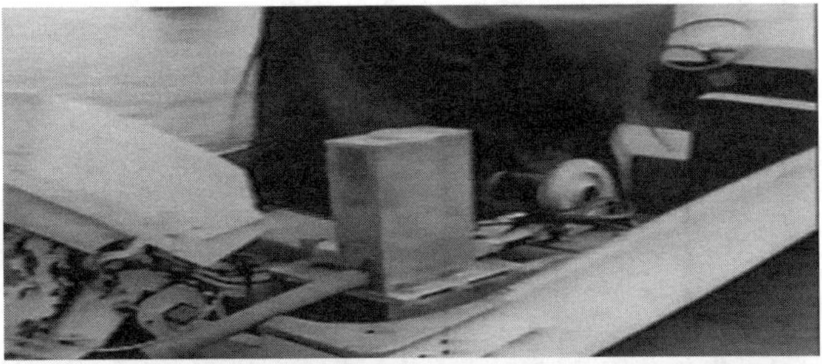

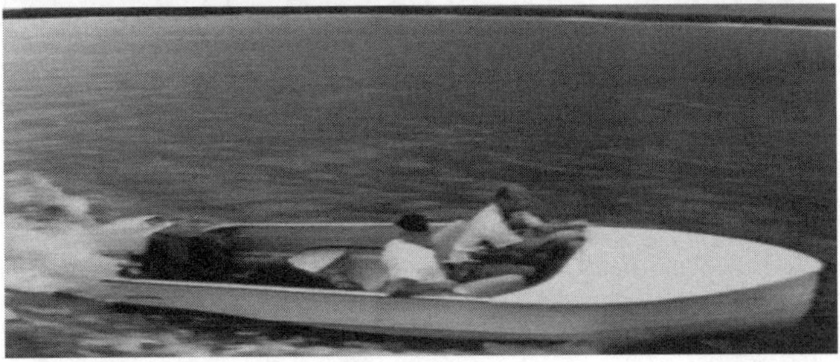

A series of field tests took place under the auspices of the U.S. Biological Laboratories from 1943 to the mid-1960s. In one such test, the cloud of simulant agent was hidden in the exhaust of an outboard boat motor. In another test, travelers at Washington National Airport were subjected to a harmless bacterium. Traps were placed throughout the facility to capture the bacterium as it flowed through the air. Laboratory personnel, dressed as travelers carrying brief cases, walked the corridors and sprayed the bacterium into the atmosphere without being detected.

1

Demented Strategies

From a military perspective, a cursory examination of the use of germs as a foundation for an effective weapon system may appear to be a good idea. Even a modest study of military history reveals that natural germ exchange at times had the effect of giving an organically robust underwhelming force a tremendous advantage during periods of conquest. The conquest of the Americas is perhaps the most seductive historical precedent capable of inspiring investigation by militaries around the world. The list of diseases introduced into the "New World" with near certainty includes smallpox and measles, and a very high probability exists that typhus, malaria, and venereal diseases should also be included. Among this list, smallpox was the greatest devastator, estimated to have killed millions as a result of the Spanish military invasion of the Americas alone.

As chronicled by the Jesuit missionaries, the Spanish military, in fact, was the first new world force to see how disease could be an ally in their imperial endeavors. The Spanish forces were small in number, but were quite successful in their conquest strategies in part due to the rampant death toll among the natives and the near incapacitation of the remainder of the resistant forces. This is not to say that the Europeans did not have problems of their own due to smallpox epidemics, but their mortality rate was much lower. Having been exposed on a regular basis to smallpox epidemics as well as to numerous other diseases acquired via natural exchanges between the Far East, Near East, North Africa, and Europe itself, the invaders had the distinct advantage of having better adapted immune systems that lowered the death toll among their populations.

In the conquest of northeastern America, the results of smallpox were predictably the same. Seemingly, there was no fatal disease to speak of in the Americas before the arrival of the Europeans, and this was noted by explorers and settlers alike. Then in 1633 an outbreak of smallpox struck New England, first laying waste the Narragansettes and the Connecticuts and then rapidly spreading into the Great Lakes Region and up the St. Lawrence River. By 1634, the Huron Indians located along the shores of Lake Ontario were deeply infected. This epidemic continued until the early 1640s and then remained relatively dormant until the 1660s. The outbreak of 1666 was particularly virulent and killed the colonists at an equally alarming rate, but as usual, it was the natives that continued to pay the heaviest price, due to shrinking populations that doomed societal survival. Cycles such as these continued well into the 18th century, and these natural catastrophes did not go unnoticed by British commanders. Sir Jeffrey Amherst (the commander of the North American British forces) suggested that smallpox be used to subdue the hostile natives of the Ohio Valley during the French and Indian Wars. When smallpox broke out at Fort Pitt, blankets and a handkerchief from the infected were collected, and on June 24, 1763, they were distributed to the natives by Captain Ecuyer. Smallpox did break out, but whether it was due to the intentional use of germs is difficult to determine, since smallpox was again breaking out all over the colonies and particularly in the Ohio Valley.

In the end, however, the deeper lesson to be learned from this series of events is that the use of germs is not a very good idea. Because of extreme collateral damage, everyone loses. In 1759, the natives gave a particularly virulent strain of smallpox to British troops in South Carolina, who in turn brought it to Charleston, thereby launching an infection rate of 75% among the population. Before long the port cities of Augusta and Savannah were also suffering from the pestilence. Looking back on these events, perhaps the most significant lesson for the military is that the advantage of a strong immune response could be capitalized upon in some way. Vaccines and germs could mean victory, but, and here is the rub, would require an astonishing tolerance for casualties.

This is not the only historical case of the use of such demented strategies. An early and profoundly significant (although potentially flawed) use of intentional germ warfare occurred at the port city of Caffa (now Feodossia, Ukraine) on the Crimean Peninsula. This Genoese colony was quite significant as a gateway to East/West trade and river trade with Russia. It had approximately 50,000 inhabitants. In 1346 an attacking "Tartar"* force (probably the Kipchak army under the subjugation of the Mongols) had this city under siege when plague broke out among its ranks. Knowing that most men died in military campaigns because of disease and that their retreat was in all probability imminent, the Tartars decided to collect their dead and catapult them over the battlements into the city. Plague broke out in Caffa, and victory became a matter of who could withstand this onslaught of disease the longest. The Tartars were victorious and chased the Italians out of the city. The colonists fled by boat to most of the major ports of Italy, and shortly thereafter plague appeared up and down the Italian coast and in Constantinople. By 1347, it was prevalent along the Mediterranean rim, and by 1348 (the standard date for the epidemic) it had spread throughout Europe. So, theoretically, began the second Black Death.

Much as with Captain Ecuyer's tactical move, we must be cautious assuming that germ warfare won the siege at Caffa, or for that matter started the second Black Death in Europe. It seems reasonable to assume that the Tartars did not understand how plague was passed along. A dead body is not as contagious as a living body. On the other hand, the handling of the corpses by people with open sores or wounds would provide an opportunity for the transmission of plague. Since "mountains of corpses" were thrown into the sea by the defenders, infection could have been passed in this manner. At the same time, while the Tartars may have been unsuccessful at breaching the walls of Caffa, rats with fleas (the primary plague vector) may have done better, so the plague could well have already been in

*This incident was a secondhand account reported by Gabriele de' Mussi.

the city. Fleas on the corpses are a much less likely source of infection. Plague-carrying fleas would typically desert a dead body and search for a living host; hence, if the bodies were not catapulted right at death or shortly thereafter, it seems unlikely that the method would work as a vector delivery system. Then again, this may have been an attempt to poison the water and torture the defenders with the relentless odor of death and not an attempt to spread plague at all. In the end, we can only say that, as an example of successful germ weaponization and deployment, this is only a plausible scenario.

Be that as it may, let us assume that the Tartars and Captain Ecuyer were successful in these early biowarfare endeavors. Between them, most problems and issues that haunt biowarfare to this day are evident: the boomerang effect, incapacitation vs. destruction of manpower, stealth, and tactical limitations. A few modern concerns are absent, such as first-strike capabilities, weapons use by those without a solid territorial affiliation, or weapons development issues. Nevertheless, the foundation for categorizing such strategies as insane by any standard of utility is readily apparent.

The Boomerang Effect Lite

While the behavior of germs is usually a subject limited to experts, the swift speed by which airborne or waterborne contagion can spread disease is a matter readily revealed by life experience, and fully recognized by the nonspecialized public. Certainly, amateur and expert alike can agree that germs do not discriminate when choosing a host (they are opportunistic) and that they do not respect national or cultural borders. Given these principles, any power seeking to weaponize these wonders of nature must consider how they can be controlled so as not to infect one's own (i.e., to prevent the germs from "boomeranging" back on friendly populations). While other matters in the weaponization process—such as the storage and distribution of virulent strains—have been optimized, and mass manufacture of virulent strains has been modernized, the issue of control has not fared as well. It seems likely that this is why various militaries have never used these weapons in combat. Given the new global order's increase in mass international travel, global shipping, and commodity exchange, the likelihood of using germ warfare without killing unintended populations is at an all-time low.

Since this problem remains unsolved, one must wonder how the research advanced at such a fast pace. During WWII and the Cold War, when bioweapons development was in full swing, the policy was much the same as that regarding nuclear power. The weapons were not developed to be used, but to deter other nations from using them. A nation showed strength by being able to render swift and devastating in-kind retaliation. For the most part, germs were not considered a first strike weapon.* One need only examine the structure of the tests done with weaponized germs to see that the militaries of the world have been, or are, quite skeptical about successfully using them.

The only recorded field tests are contested, although it seems probable that in October and November 1940 the Japanese made

*During the 1950s the United States flirted with the idea that the use of germs for purposes of incapacitation could be a conventional offensive weapon and not one of mass destruction.

three attempts to air drop plague-contaminated fleas and other assorted materials such as wheat and rice (presumably to attract rats) on towns in China. Each time one of these odd bombing runs were made, plague broke out. The cities struck were Chuhsien, Ningpo, and Kinhwa. None of these cities had the facilities to culture the bacteria that may have been in the fleas, so a direct link between the fleas and the plague outbreaks could not be established with certainty. The casualties were minimal.

The Japanese did try one last field test in October 1941, but after the initial drops, their policy changed, and instead they began testing in labs or in more secluded areas. It is possible that the Japanese were simply unhappy with the results. In interviews conducted by Murray Sanders at the Dai-Ichi building with Ishii Shiro, the head of Japan's biowarfare program, Ishii said that fleas could not be successfully dropped from airplanes. Instead, Ishii went on to experiment with anthrax and anthrax delivery systems—most notably developing a kind of biocluster bomb called the Uji bomb.

One important early successful scientific test of germ weapons was done by the British on Gruinard Island off the coast of Scotland. This is a remote location, to say the least, and was known in the Ministry of Defense as X Base. On July 15, 1942, a thirty-pound bomb loaded with anthrax suspension was dropped from a gallows. The test subjects were a herd of sheep, and the purpose of the test was to see how effective an anthrax bomb would be with suitable air currents. The test was for inhalation contamination only. The sheep were placed in crates and their heads placed in canvas hoods so they could not lick any spores off their bodies. Of the fifteen sheep in the herd only two survived—those furthest away from the blast. Blood smears were taken from each of the dead sheep in order to be sure they had died of anthrax. The test was repeated, resulting in a slightly poorer kill ratio, but this was due to an unexpected shift in wind direction. (This is a good example of how, even under the best conditions, the weapons can function in unexpected ways.) The next test consisted of a bomb dropped from an airplane, which failed because the bomb landed in a peat bog and sank. The experiment was moved to another remote location on the coast of Wales. The bombing was a success, disproving the theory that no anthrax could survive a bomb explosion. While it was estimated that 90% of the anthrax was killed in the explosion, the remaining 10% did provide the desired result, with a 90% mortality rate. However, this result could not be consistently repeated.

In April 1979, the Soviet biowarfare unit Compound 19 at Sverdlovsk (home to a large-scale military weapons manufacturing site and a city of 1.2 million people, now known as Yekaterinaburg) noticed that a neighboring population was experiencing a serious outbreak of anthrax. Soviet émigrés to Germany told local newspapers that the factory had released a cloud of anthrax spores. What actually happened is uncertain. Seemingly, 66 deaths occurred in a 4-km swath downwind from the incident. The United States military and various intelligence corps believed that an anthrax aerosol was accidentally released. Further evidence came from satellite images of roadblocks and what appeared to be decontamination trucks in the area. Later, Soviet doctors who were involved in the event came forward saying that it was an accident and published details of victim autopsies. The official Soviet claim was that the deaths were due to a batch of anthrax-tainted meat that unfortunately was distributed in the town. Whatever the truth may be, the newly elected Reagan administration capitalized on this situation by using it as an example of why its suggested multi-trillion dollar military buildup should be accepted by government and citizens alike.

The Soviets got more than they bargained for. Not only did they have a public relations disaster, scores of dead citizens, and a contamination that would be quite costly to clean up, but they were also saddled with an intensification of the arms race. They had unwittingly contributed to a paranoid American fantasy engine that in turn led to more spending on useless technology. The boomerang could work on two fronts—not just militarily, but on the collective imagination and ideological order as well.

A Brief Word on Kill Ratios and Tacticality

Another lesson can be learned from all the above examples. The Japanese, the Soviets, and the British agreed on one thing—anthrax is the germ of choice for warfare. Anthrax minimizes the boomerang effect since it cannot be spread from person to person like plague or smallpox. In addition, it can be transformed into "spores." In this dormant form, it is incredibly resistant to heat, drying, and sunlight, which means it is compatible with missile or bomb deployment systems and can be used for daylight attack. Anthrax is relatively easy to make, and it can be made quite virulent. It appears to be the perfect weapon, but how dependable is its mortality rate? The British experiments indicated an incredibly high kill ratio in the first test; however, this occurred under perfect meteorological conditions in a controlled environment. The failure of the second test, in which wind shifted, is indicative of the weapon's poor dependability.

The Soviets did not do as well with their accidental test. Only 66 deaths occurred in a heavily populated area in which the inhabitants were completely unaware of the accident. From a military perspective, this number cannot be too impressive. Any other weapon of mass destruction and most conventional weapons would prove more deadly. To the contrary, the World Heath Organization claims that 50 kg of *B. anthracis* released in a population center of 500,000 would deliver 95,000 deaths and 125,000 incapacitations (these are the kinds of figures that the military and publicly funded institutions presented to Congress in connection with germ warfare). These numbers could only be derived from a simulation, unlike the Soviet experience with actual field conditions. While the attack could possibly be improved by planned use of meteorological conditions, it remains unlikely that this would radically change the scenario.

Even under optimum conditions, germs are relatively useless as a tactical weapon. Their efficiency is questionable, and they are dependent on unstable conditions such as the weather. The last thing any military person wants is a weapon that needs help from entropic nature to have a chance at performing well. Such a weapon could, on the other hand, be used in ventilation systems where the air currents are more predictable and reliable. The stealth advantage of using tasteless, odorless, invisible germs is worth considering in the indoor scenario; however, why a military would want to employ a weapon of random death that would be limited to a single building is hard to imagine. Only under rare conditions would there be a military advantage, and for terrorists, more profoundly symbolic and terrible ways to kill are just as available. This leaves the subway, where an attack could potentially go on for days before anyone would know (alert to the attack would only come after numerous people started showing symptoms) and infect who knows how many people. A simulation of a NYC subway anthrax attack done in the 1960s indicated approximately 10,000 deaths would occur if the release were done at rush hour. Perhaps the underground is anthrax's tactical *raison d'etre* for those interested in civilian targets. On the other hand, such a weapon would fail to destroy this valuable piece of infrastructure.

Strategic Germ Warfare

For the United States and seemingly for the major military powers of the world, the use of germ warfare, like the use of any weapon of mass destruction, is typically for strategic purposes. They are all used for purposes of deterrence. The theory is that a hostile state recognizes that if any attack with a weapon of mass destruction is perpetrated on the home state or its allies, an increasingly devastating, in-kind reprisal will be the reward. (This is not to say that the United States military has not and is not developing tactical and offensive weapons. It certainly is, but these are weapon systems that it is in no hurry to use.) The function of these weapons is to act as a material grounding for the manufacture of an exchangeable sign of maximum threat. Among major military powers, this sign must indicate that no advantage or reward can be gained by the use of the weapons. Generally, this form of military neutralization is taken to an extreme in the form of a policy of mutually assured destruction. From a greater power to a lesser power, the sign must indicate that use of such weapons will only bring disadvantage, since the power of the greater military is understood to be overwhelmingly superior. And from a lesser power to a greater power, the sign must say that this force is capable of inflicting severe casualties, so that while this force might be defeated, its enemies will pay a very heavy cost.

CAE now is compelled to ask: From a military perspective, when does strategic deterrence with weapons of mass destruction (WMD) become counterproductive? We believe that even within the logic of the military itself, germ warfare is not useful. Assuming, as the military does, that WMDs are a self-evident aspect of postmodern war and that deterrence is a successful strategy for coping with this element of warfare, what use do germs really have? For major military powers, they would seem to offer very little. They are not very effective field weapons compared to other WMDs (nuclear, chemical, and poison), so they offer no specialized function that any other WMD couldn't provide with more desirable results. Among equals, their only uses are as a modest mutual logistical drain and as a means to create additional threat intensities. These weapons are not something minor powers must concern themselves with developing. Such weapons would not be used against them except as a retaliatory response, making the logistical advantage moot in these situations (i.e., they don't have to keep up with the Joneses since minor powers are not a part of strategic play). Further, since there have been no hot clashes between major powers since World War II, having a variety of WMDs seems to be wasteful and very poor planning for the types of wars that are likely to be fought. Isn't having just one type of WMD (nuclear being the most effective) enough to maintain a deterrence policy? For WMDs, it is only the retaliatory results that matter (mutually assured destruction). Such results only require the most effective weapon systems.

Must a military power respond in kind to a WMD? This seems to be a piece of conventional wisdom that has not been considered for some time. The belief that a state must retaliate with the same WMD has little to do with military efficiency and more to do with response from other states. (Again, any WMD that is effective should do the job.) The fear is that a different WMD will expand the theater of usage and draw condemnation from allies. However, because we have not seen this situation since the world wars, we have no contemporary example of state-against-state use of WMDs to judge this wisdom (with perhaps the exception of defoliant in Vietnam). But if we take WWI as the best historical example, the hope for successful limited use of WMDs once any are used is quite vain (they will all be used), so a retaliating force may as well use what works best.

Returning to the subject of logistical drain, germs are at the bottom of the hierarchy of utility. If the military learned anything during Reagan's military buildup during the Cold War, it is that war must be expensive. (This was a policy suggested by antigerm warfare scientist Matthew S. Meselson while consulting on matters of germ warfare during the Kennedy administration.*)

---

*Meselson was a Harvard biologist who denounced the use of germ warfare throughout the 1960s to both the Kennedy and Nixon administrations. His pleas were ignored by Kennedy, primarily because too much money had already been invested in the germ warfare program, thus making it difficult to tell the public how useless it was. Meselson consulted for Nixon at the request of former Harvard colleague Henry Kissinger. In 1969 Meselson wrote a paper for the White House on the uselessness of germ warfare. Nixon, unlike Kennedy, listened (although more likely as a means to deflect criticism over his Vietnam policy than due to Meselson's arguments) and began to organize the 1972/75 biological weapons ban treaty.

The more expensive it is to prepare and wage a war, the better. As Paul Virilio has shown in *Pure War*, logistics are the key to a successful postmodern war.

Even for a state that is economically and militarily small, germs are cheap to manufacture, so if there is a desire to go this route, it is possible. The major powers have tried to increase the cost by developing a soft international consensus that disallows minor military powers from having WMDs. This means that minor powers with military ambitions are put in the position of being stealthy enough with WMD programs that no state can prove they have them, but transparent enough that the weapons can be used strategically as a potential threat. However, this added cost does not put the manufacture of military grade germs out of reach. The real problem for a minor power is that a war will in all probability be fought on its own territory (a minor power does not have a global military) and that would be the last place any force would want to spread germs. Since offensive delivery systems are very expensive to manufacture and maintain, no minor power has the means to attack a major power on its home turf other than in very limited forms that only earn them a devastating response. To complicate matters further, if we look at the example of the first Gulf War, the chemical/germ deterrence strategy did not work very well. On the other hand, North Korea chose nuclear weapons as a deterrent and has fared better, judging by the degree of caution that has been shown by capitalist powers. In this case, a "diplomatic solution" appears to be the chosen option. This proven Cold War strategy consists of an effort to bankrupt the enemy state through economic isolation combined with internal economic pressures stemming from the staggering cost of maintaining a standing army. Once this is accomplished, the hope is that the "rogue" state will come to the bargaining table or that the government will be toppled by friendlier internal forces.

Based on experience, as opposed to nightmare scenarios dreamed up by those who desire a fully militarized state, germ warfare is a waste, a burning excess that in the end does little more than terrorize a nation's own citizenry. Is it surprising that even the U.S. declared "madman" Saddam Hussein did not use biological weapons (if indeed he had them) during either of the Gulf Wars? Obviously not. For nations and other territorialized groups, biological weapons are more of a burden and a sign of threat that is easily erased.

Bioterrorism

If the thesis is accepted that germ-based weapon systems have a very limited tactical and strategic capacity for nations, and because of this, the probability of them ever being used is quite low, we must ask who would find this poor man's weapon desirable? The threat makers and fear mongers are very quick to answer that terrorists will want to use them! For most of the groups that one or more nations have labeled as terrorist organizations, the probability of this happening is again very low. The reason is that most of these groups are locked in a territorialized struggle for self-determination in which WMDs are not of any strategic or tactical use. Whether one examines the examples of terrorist organizations in Spain, Northern Ireland, Palestine, Sri Lanka, East Timor, etc., they all share one commonality—that for these struggles to achieve a goal of landed autonomy, they must court positive support from the international community as well as support from the local citizenry. International support is necessary to pressure the dominant power to negotiate, and if that is successful, to mediate these negotiations, while the local citizenry must be supportive enough (and exhausted enough) to put internal pressure on the government to do what is necessary to resolve the situation. Since the international community has defined the use of WMDs as an intolerable "crime against humanity," no territorialized resistance movement of self-determination can afford to so deeply offend those they need help from, and worse, essentially give their opponent the opportunity to "justly" respond to their criminal action by whatever means they may choose. It should be remembered these are rational struggles that have clear and possible objectives and only the instruments that serve these objectives will be employed.

But what about the small minority of terrorist organizations that are not territorialized, find transnational solidarity in some type of religious fundamentalism, and have strong eschatological values? From the perspective of pancapitalism, these groups have regard neither for material accumulation nor humanitarian principles, and thereby can only be understood as nonrational forces of negation bent on destruction. Whether this portrait is fair or accurate is another subject, but this representation enjoys a tremendous amount of exchange and convinces the United States authorities that a major attack is "not a matter of if, but when." In this category of organizations, we can be certain there is one organization willing to cause mass civilian casualties, and that is al Qaeda. We can also be certain the weapons they have used thus far, while odd, are conventional. As for the use of germs in particular, since their fight is transnational, and since potentially a sympathizer has already used them (in the October 2001 anthrax attack in the United States), it is possible that such weapons would be used if they could acquire them. However, this possibility needs to be put in perspective. Acquisition of the germs on a large scale would be difficult at best, and it is even less likely that the organization could produce them internally given the incredible military pressure it is under. Germ production is neither common among guerrillas roaming the mountains of Pakistan and Afghanistan, nor among sleeper cells trying to maintain deep cover. Could a sympathizer in medical research supply the necessary material? Yes, but only for a small tactical operation. No medical researchers can lay their hands on 50 kgs of untraceable anthrax, especially in the United States with its new, ultra-sensitive security measures. A small tactical strike is not very destructive, and in spite of all the hoopla from the only germ attack so far, the casualties were tragic, but minimal. Planes and boxcutters were much more effective.

Germ attacks are too rare to be taken so seriously. In the United States there have only been three other incidents of germ terrorism coming from the nonterritorialized transnational terrorists. Two were from fascist groups. In 1972, members of the Order of the Rising Sun were found in possession of approximately 35 kgs of typhoid bacteria cultures with which they were planning to poison the water supply in Chicago and St. Louis. They were arrested before they could execute the plan. The second incident occurred in 1995, when Larry Wayne Harris of the Aryan Nation attempted to purchase three vials of freeze-dried bubonic plague from American Type Culture Collection. Harris was arrested before he received the vials.

The best-known case (besides the anthrax attack) occurred in The Dalles, Oregon when members of the Rajaneeshee cult grew a strain of Salmonella and deployed it in restaurant salad bars around the area. There were approximately 750 incapacitations, 45 hospitalizations, and zero deaths. They purchased the bacteria from American Type Culture Collection for their medical center, so no suspicions were raised, and it was only due to a schism within the power structure of the cult that the plan was revealed. What was particularly odd about this attack was their motivation. They were not bent on destruction but were attempting to rig local elections by incapacitating the citizens who would vote against their candidates.

It appears to CAE that funneling more funds into germ warfare research and extreme overpreparedness when there is only the modest chance of a germ attack is a terrible waste of public funds. These funds would be better used trying to defeat diseases such as malaria and HIV that prematurely end the lives of millions of people every year. The military has consistently shown its ability to embrace waste and uselessness, and even claims that these unconscionable expenditures are a strategic benefit. However, when this is done at the expense of public health, this form of sacrificial economy cannot be allowed to continue. Not since the 1960s has there been significant pressure from citizen groups and scientific professionals to end germ warfare programs. As we shall show in upcoming chapters, we do not need more preparedness, nor are the treaties that supposedly limit these programs actually working. Much as during the Cold War, this moment of hypercapital expenditure in favor of expanding the war machine is as difficult to intervene in as it is to effectively support robust public health and health care for all.

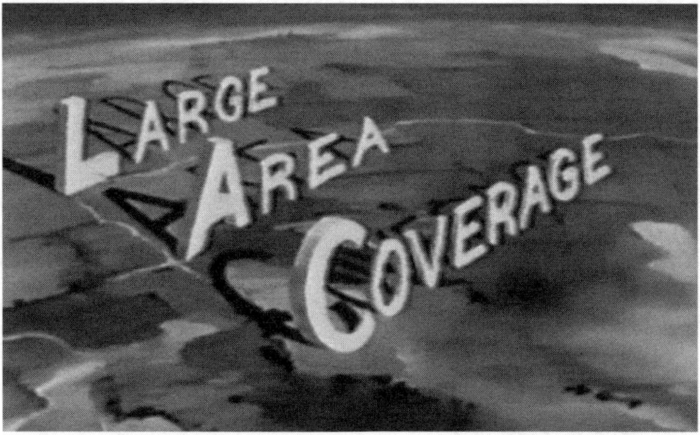

Other tests performed as part of the U.S. offensive biological weapons program include:

In San Francisco, a U.S. Navy ship equipped with spray devices operated by Fort Detrick personnel sprayed Serratia marcescens, a non-pathogenic microorganism that is easily detected, while the ship plied the San Francisco Bay. It spread more than 30 miles to monitoring stations.

A jet aircraft equipped with spray devices flew a course near Victoria, Texas, and the harmless particles were monitored in the Florida Keys.

2

Circuits of the Plague

The currency may be different within each of the power vectors able to capitalize on the threat of germ warfare, but payday has arrived, and the best part is that claiming a reward only requires the appearance of productivity. Votes for politicians, viewers and readers for the media, research funds for Big Science and Medicine, a vastly expanding budget for the military, and perhaps most importantly, the consolidation of power for the dominant political party are all on the table, and the various institutions able to gain from these rewards are already counting their riches. Any self-respecting capitalist institution should be able to exploit this false economy of threat, but it must follow one simple rule: it must agree to expanded militarization of its resources and its relations to its particular form of production. This is not to say that all civil functions must be eliminated; it is only to say that more tribute (perhaps more than ever before) must be paid to the sacrificial economy of the military. Any enterprise that accomplishes this task is welcome, and the tribute may be paid in symbolic or material form. Manufacturing or maintaining the public perception of imminent biological threat or militarizing civil process are both acceptable forms of payment that double as a means to profit for the broad variety of confederates.

While the circuit of exchange is grander than it has ever been, this model of opportunity in relation to biothreat dates back to the 1930s. At that time, the idea of maximizing profit and consolidating power through the matrix of biocatastrophe was launched. One might be tempted to think this was an idea that had to originate in the United States where the arms industry was at full tilt following the boom of sales to Europe during World War I, but this is not the case. The United States military, at this point in time, did not see much value in germ warfare, nor had it yet assumed the policy of weaponizing any material or process that could be weaponized. Instead, this idea found a responsive state in imperial Japan, and Ishii Shiro, a major in the Army Medical Corps, was the mastermind who developed it.

Ishii's inspiration was threefold in nature: an encephalitis outbreak in Shikoku, the 1925 Geneva protocol, and his own practical work for the Japanese military. In 1930, Ishii was working at the Tokyo Army Medical College. During this time, he developed a ceramic filter that could eliminate bacteria and viruses from water. Given the imperial ambitions of Japan, the military situated itself in many tropical territories where waterborne disease was an extreme hazard. His invention was seen as a miracle breakthrough. The filter was adopted by both the Army and Navy, and Ishii was handsomely rewarded with royalties from the use of the device. For this work, he not only received a substantial fortune, he also gained legitimacy in the eyes of the state. When it came to policy regarding disease, Ishii was a man to consult and listen to. He clearly knew that aiding the military in defending against germs was a fast track to wealth and power, and he had no trouble making the jump to exploring the use of germs for military advantage as a means to achieve the same results.

His first consideration of germs as a weapon probably dates back to his experience of the encephalitis outbreak on the island of Shikoku in 1924. The disease and how it spread (via mosquitoes) was not known until much later, and while Ishii could not do anything to stem the rate of infection, he did get to see just how devastating a contagion like this could be. In all, 3,500 people died of severe brain inflammation. Considering the Geneva Protocol of 1925 (Japan did not sign until 1970), Ishii reasoned that elimination of the use of "bacteriological methods of warfare" would only be done if the various militaries of the world considered dangerous strains of bacteria to be effective, useful weapons. These thoughts and experiences led him to give a series of lectures in 1931 on the advantages of weaponizing germs. As a fully legitimized, well connected, medical microbiologist, Ishii commanded the authority to make his new scheme a reality. After all, no one doubted that germs were effective killers that had brought many an army to the point of ruin. For example, the destruction of Justinian's seemingly undefeatable army during the first Black Death in Europe would make any military mind at least consider the idea. Ishii was also quite a showman, and he understood the value of a good performance even if the facts of the matter had to be bent a little. Ishii told the Imperial Command that the Russians were using germ warfare in Manchuria and the Chinese were poisoning wells with cholera. None of these claims was ever substantiated, and in all probability they were not true, but it did not matter. The Japanese army was fully convinced, and in 1932 awarded Ishii the resources he needed. This included a research lab at the Army Medical College in Tokyo, a bacterial production facility in Harbin, China, and a test site close to the facility in Beiyinhe.

By 1940, now Major-General Ishii was at the peak of his power. His facility at Ping Fan was a modern marvel in regard to germ warfare. It was called the Anti-Epidemic Water Supply and Purification Bureau. Within the 150 buildings on the site there were labs, autopsy rooms, a bombing test site, and a bacteria culture plant. When running at full speed, this plant could produce a monthly yield of 300 kgs of plague organisms, 500 kgs of anthrax spores, or 1,000 kgs of cholera. Ishii had 3,000 workers under his command, and the site provided adequate housing, an independent power plant, and a farm to help them along. He also offered recreational facilities for the workers, including a library, a 1,000-seat theater, restaurants, an athletic field, a swimming pool, and even a brothel.

Ishii had carved a mini empire for himself by selling his idea of germ warfare. However, in spite of these grand resources, his program was fundamentally useless. Nothing it produced was ever successfully used in a military campaign. A method to successfully deploy his weapons was never devised. His few field tests were either inconclusive, or killed as many Japanese troops as they did Russians or Chinese. (Whether Ishii's weapons caused plague and cholera in Northern Manchuria is difficult to know, because these diseases were already active in the region and could have spread simply as a byproduct of army life.) He never got even the symbolic benefits of the germ threat since the program was kept secret and was not discovered by the allies until 1944. By 1942, Ishii's program was doing little more than eating away at Japan's dwindling resources, although he did continue to produce a lot of flash (the Uji bomb for example) and hype. Unfortunately, the useless nature of Ishii's program was not its legacy, rather it is the flash that lives on. From a present day perspective, Ishii's brilliance was not his idea for germ warfare, but his recognition of the opportunity to create wealth and power for himself by capitalizing on the fear of germs and their destructive power.

Opportunity for the military state is presenting itself again. The clear and obvious place is in the vast expansion of military budgets in general and of germ warfare programs in particular. The armed forces of the United States may once again gorge themselves on a never-ending supply of resources. They may pursue any fancy no matter how demented, useless, or impossible it may be. These obese vampires can bleed the public dry as long as "security" remains the priority issue and as long as the hyperreality of threat can sustain itself in the imagination of the grand majority of citizens. However, more is at stake than just funds. The military state now sees the opportunity to expand its domain over the civil sector—centering itself as the most important consideration in any economic or political process. The agencies that enable movement, such as the government, the media, science, and medicine are also targets for increased endo-colonization by the military; however, their complicity will earn them a share of the profits of threat.

The Security Industry

Anyone who has visited an airport recently has not only witnessed, but has experienced the spectacle and reality of security intensification—not that it is so much more efficient than it used to be. Other than more ID checks, spiffier uniforms for the security agents, the x-raying of shoes, and the prohibition of visitors at the departure gates, it's basically the same as it always was. Most activities are only there to create the appearance of a secure space, to make travelers less anxious, and to show their tax dollars are at work making everyone a little safer. Actually, this spectacle is a huge waste of taxpayer dollars; passengers were just as safe with the old system. All that really needed to be modified was to prohibit box cutters and related items on the plane and to secure the pilot's cabin door. Surely the former airport employees could have coped with these small adjustments. But there are more interesting proposals on the table than the immediately visible make-work initiative for the feds: The real question seems to be, "How do we make the transportation industry more like the security industry?" After all, the environment is perfect. Visibility is great, people are used to a strict authoritarian environment, and there is relative assurance as to who each individual is. This is the kind of situation that makes police work easy. The problem is that the airline industry is not a police force. However, this problem is being solved through synergistic application. For example, why can't a database of those with outstanding warrants be linked to passenger databases? Such a practice would insure safer flights *and* get criminals off the street. Or, why can't the Homeland Security terrorist watch list be linked to passenger databases? Seemingly a good idea, except for the fact that Homeland Security is very generous in who it places on the list (even your humble authors are on the list). The generality, not the particularity, is really what is so undesirable. The prevailing logic is that all civilian industry should have dual function—its service or manufacturing function and its security function. Not only that, all travelers should now be police. In a stunning reversal of policy, travelers are encouraged not to cooperate with a hijacker and to fight back. After all, the hijacker is going to kill all the passengers anyway. Is it any wonder that xenophobic vigilante activity is breaking out all over the United States and particularly on the border with Mexico? The policing model we now find in airports and the premises that underlie it are cornerstones in the foundation of a police state.

On July 7, 2005, the security state was given another gift with the bombings of the subway and a bus in London. The question they brought forth was, "Why should the airport model not be expanded to all forms of public transportation?" The subways of most major cities became immediate military zones complete with police gangs conducting "random" searches. The subway offers the state the benefit of reaching far more people than the airports and apparently with little resistance thus far. CAE cannot demonstrate that the searches are not random, or that they are an abuse of power (there have been no studies yet). However, we can impressionistically say, based on our own experience on a watch list, there are two scenarios that launch a search. One, a person is on a watch list, or two, a person is profiled. From our long experience with secondary customs, CAE would like to reassure right wing bigots everywhere that a policy of profiling is what is being enacted even if it is not the official policy. Every time we have been in secondary customs, we have been there solely with Arab peoples. At the subway, this base can expand as police use their new mandate to protect to profile for drugs and guns as well as terrorists. What demographic would the police think has drugs and guns?

The airport/subway militarization is revealing in other ways as well. The United States is beginning to pay more attention to police methodology by following the example of its ally, the United Kingdom. While the United States has always had an approach to policing based in presence (the cop on the beat) and showing their colors whenever and wherever possible, the British have preferred a virtual style of policing. Let the cameras do the walking. Everything from robbery to speeding tickets is primarily policed via cameras. Now for the United States, the course of action is clear: use it all. People are already used to being on camera all the time and no longer think about it as an invasion of privacy. Like taxes, surveillance is just a fact of life. The possibility that U.S. systems will become as advanced as those used in London's financial district (where everyone is scanned upon entering and a criminal data base is consulted to see if any match occurs) appears increasingly likely given the latest trends.

Bentham's panopticon, found in so much prison architecture, is now little more than alibi for the illusion that whatever may pass for public or private space is not a panoptic architecture. The panopticon is the Disneyland of post 9/11 society—a place to see incarceration as a display, whether it is Joliet or Camp X-Ray that is being viewed and virtualized. Indeed, one of the security state's greatest achievements is its new line of prisons. The national prison system becomes a mere byproduct of modern capitalism and of the nostalgia for slavery. The new prisons, in all their glorious absence, offer the security state more than just a means of prison industry expansion—they offer new types of authoritarian power. Most are quite apparent, and CAE won't belabor them. The clearest lesson from Gitmo is that anyone can be held without legal consultation or due process. Abu Ghraib has shown the world the latest in torture techniques. And then, there are the secret prisons. What happens to all the enemy prisoners that the news tells the American public about each day? They just disappear. A policy of secrecy and darkness exists, a true favorite of the United States in its overseas activities.

Here is where surveillance gets interesting. While most critics concerned with surveillance focus on capital's peeking and processing capabilities in relation to the fate of an increasingly illuminated global citizenry, they too often forget about the territories and populations that are off the panoptic grid. The United States does its part well in dispensing deillumination privileges—plenty of cells in the world panopticon have a legitimized lights out. The power of darkness is not just a characteristic of the central watch tower, but occurs in all the cells of those who are the trustees of capital. For example, information on the treatment of the Kurds (both civilian/refugees and insurgents) by the Turkish military is rather scarce and must be actively searched for. When Iraq ferociously attacked the Kurds with a variety of weapons (including chemical ones), that was bad behavior but tolerable, because Hussein was still an ally in the initiative to undermine Iran. During the Gulf War, however, the atrocities against the Kurds were intolerable, and the invisible Kurds lost in darkness were returned to the light and protected in Northern Iraq. But not in Turkey: that situation is still in blackout conditions, and the United States is still willing to supply whatever arms are needed to keep the blood flowing. The same privileges of deillumination are granted to (just to name a few) Indonesia, Israel, Saudi Arabia, and until recently even the Taliban. These regimes seem to be able to make whatever trouble they want in their darkened cells, as long as they do not act contrary to the interests of the watchers.

Another interrelated place in the cultural terrain is the internal attack on dissenting voices within the U.S. citizenry, or even worse, in order to create an internal enemy, on those whose only "crime" is being of the Islamic faith. The Department of Justice has realized that it can expand its power base by finding ways to classify citizens as enemy combatants. The most horrific case is still that of the Lackawana Six, which according to President Bush represented a successful busting of a "sleeper cell." Prior to 9/11, six Yemeni teens went to Afghanistan to study the Koran. While there, they found themselves at an al Qaeda training camp, which they left as quickly as they could. They returned to the United States and resumed their usual routines. After 9/11, the FBI discovered they had attended this camp and saw that as an excuse to raid the entire Yemeni community–kicking in doors and forcing innocent people out of their homes. The six boys who went to Afghanistan were all arrested. The boys were told by the Justice Department that if they did not plead guilty to material support of terrorism, they would be reclassified as enemy combatants and shipped off to Guantanamo. Having few resources at their disposal, the boys were intimidated into taking the deal. The prosecuting attorney, William Hochul (who is also prosecuting your humble authors), has since admitted that he had no evidence that these boys were doing anything other than living a lawful existence.

Clearly, the security state is spreading like a virus throughout the United States and, unfortunately, with the blessings of those who would sacrifice their own autonomy and their own interests for a feeling of security. If this is a virus of everyday life, one can only imagine the relation of the security state to the production of knowledge that has economic and military application. The life sciences are being militarized through the use of the carrot and the stick. Oddly enough, one division of the life sciences that was nearly in the grave in terms of the generation of breakthrough knowledge, microbiology, is back from the brink. Not because it will generate anything new and amazing, but because the government and military need to know about germs in general and how the military could use them in particular. The money is flowing, but, with government money, there is always a catch. The investment must be secure. For businesses, this is not a problem as the two have a common interest in keeping what they know private and secure and in that they share an authoritarian micro-culture. For universities, the problem is unmanageable, since the university is charged with producing public, not private, knowledge. Its mandate is to contribute to the cultural commons for the educational good of all. Unfortunately, the cultural commons as a territory of knowledge production is a high priority target for the security state. Knowledge is not for free thinking, but for the instrumental task of advancing the interests of the investing classes. From the perspective of the security state, all knowledge having to do with profit or violence should be privatized and distributed on a need-to-know basis.

The means by which movement is made toward this goal varies. For universities with little money, the offer of funding is simply an easy bribe. For those universities with excess cash resources, the promise of a flagship project is necessary. The real bribe here is not money and equipment, but prestige. This type of bribery as a form of knowledge control is very broad-based. Within the life sciences, the usual suspects of genetics, molecular biology, and microbiology are not the only ones in on the germ warfare big bonanza: botany, zoologogy, and environmental biology can also get a piece of the pie. (The National Institute of Allergy and Infectious Diseases has recommended that as many of the sciences as possible be brought into the germ warfare family. Most of these nontraditional members are coming in through the Biowatch program and are involved in creating sentinel organisms). Once inside, the security state equips all doors with locks to keep out any trespassers. Any type of amateur, any colleague not on the project, any interdisciplinarian, or any student must be kept outside, because they have no justification for access to this knowledge and are a potential security threat. Those locked inside are subject to security review, their protocols are policed, and they must be silent about their work—a very bad situation for pedagogues, but not much better for the janitors. Here lies the second cornerstone of the police state—privatize and lock down knowledge. Given the current intensity of these "security" tendencies, this nation can only be politically classified as proto-fascist.

Politics and Plague

One unfortunate irony floating through U.S. politics is that when the public hears White House spokespeople on the evening agitprop report say, "We are winning the war on terrorism," they are hearing the truth, but misinterpreting it. The two common interpretive positions are the White House is telling us the plain truth, or the White House is lying and the United States and its allies are actually losing; i.e., the insurgency is growing in Iraq, and terrorism is expanding in Europe with no end in site. The problem is that both interpretations of the statement are wrong. The confusion stems from the use of the word "we." Many citizens are deluded into thinking the "we" includes them. It does not. In this case of meta-irony, or irony squared, "we" means authoritarian power vectors (APVs), and "winning" means coming to power. While the terrorists are in conflict with the APVs, the APVs find the situation to be in harmony with their interests.

The goal of terrorism is not military victory, but a negotiated settlement. To meet this objective, acts of terror are perpetrated with the goal of getting an extreme reaction out of the government attacked. If these attacks are sustained over a long period of time (decades if necessary) and the government under attack continues to take a reactionary position,* an authoritarian state will emerge that will exploit and torment the citizenry in the same manner as it does the culture represented by the terrorists (or as they consider themselves, freedom fighters). Once the citizens are so enlightened, as well as being tired of the ongoing attacks, they will pressure for negotiations from the inside. In this case, fundamentalist extremists carrying out the recent terrorist attacks worldwide believe that the West is a colonial army occupying their land, attempting to dictate cultural policy

---

* Spain, a far more committed democracy than the United States, refused to take a reactionary position in regard to terrorism or to move into a state of security panic. The experience and maturity gained through the struggle with Basque separatists is revealed in investigative and defense initiatives that reflect an understanding of terrorist strategy, as well as terrorism's relation to duration.

and stealing or exploiting economic resources. This same set of conditions (but in endocolonial form) is what they hope to bring to the West, believing that the citizens of a democracy will never tolerate such a situation and would rather see their diplomats negotiate for an honorable peace. In the majority of cases in the West, this assumption is appropriate, but in the case of the United States, it could not be more inappropriate. The conditions that the extremists want to produce are the very conditions desired by APVs. Rather than fighting the United States, the terrorists are actually contributing to the dominant general political goal—a full-scale authoritarian government. They are sadly mistaken if they think they will get anywhere with this strategy, since the United States will only too gladly intensify its endo-authoritarian tendencies in the belief that once the citizens wake up to what they have lost, it will be too late—authoritarian structure will have solidified.

The problem U.S. proto-fascists have is that the terrorists are not fulfilling their end of the bargain. Since 9/11, there has not been any activity in the United States. Because the terrorists are so slow (getting a powerful attack going about every ten years), the current right-wing government itself has to terrorize the citizens. One of its favorite topics to fall back on is bioterrorism. What would happen if we were attacked? In Chapter One, CAE showed that a large-scale attack is nearly an impossibility. The staged drills in major cities, the stockpiling of vaccines, the emotional calls for increased attention to this hazard, and most importantly the announcement by Secretary of Homeland Security Michael Chertoff that bioterrorism is on the top priority list of major concerns—all are performed to keep the fear level high. The key here is for politicians to look like they are doing something that responds to the concerns of a given constituency. If the constituents are concerned about bioterrorism and nothing is happening, it is incumbent upon their representatives to make something happen in order to simulate doing something about the crisis that doesn't exist. The spectacle is as significant as the real. Body invasion and nuclear holocaust are the best provocateurs as weapons of mass distraction, and they are being called upon with ritualistic regularity. Luckily for the government, the media has never met a weapon of mass distraction that it did not like.

News Media, Threat, and Profit

On the one hand, the media has long had a conflicted relationship with state and corporate power. Even the most respected particular forms such as journalism and news reporting have had to pay tribute to their news providers (the state and military). These payments tend to conflict, sometimes bitterly, with the more idealistic goals of neutral observation and objective fact-based reporting. On the other hand, a conflict with its audience also exists. The viewers have to want to watch or read the reportage and this constitutes another pressure that must be addressed. Caught between these two pressures, the media industry in general and the news media in particular are in the unfortunate practical position of having to negotiate this problem of truth-bending demands while attempting to best approximate their ideals. In order to optimize this situation, the news media prefer it when the two forces can be made complementary to one another; i.e., when what the state wants to tell the media audience is what the audience wants to hear. One of the most dependable narratives used to create this dovetail effect is that of crisis. The crisis narrative generates a fear that something bad could happen to the individual or to valued resources that individuals want. In turn, a desire emerges for preparedness (or knowledge of preparation by a protectorate) that will return the general audience to a state of security. Information about how to regain a state of relative calm comes from the state, relayed by the media. In this scenario, everyone gets what s/he wants. The state gets its position communicatively exchanged as a necessary legitimized fact; the media attracts motivated viewers, satisfying advertisers and investors and thus increasing its profit potential; and the audience gets information about the crisis, along with a "reassuring" promise that the crisis is being engaged and neutralized.

In spite of this trajectory of cooperation, the news media have the problem of maintaining the journalistic integrity that enables the public perception of legitimacy in regard to the reporting of facts. In addition, the perception of crisis must be maintained, and facts often get in the way of this narrative promotion. To evade the reporting of facts that could disrupt the representation desired by the state, as much time as possible is spent on nonfactual discussion. Experts, consultants, and editorialists are enlisted to wildly speculate on the apocalyptic outcomes of a given crisis scenario and to talk about what could be done to circumvent these outcomes. Such discussions reinforce the appearance of the crisis as immediate and undeniable, while at the same time creating both a discourse of preparedness that can function in the interest of the state and military and a representational environment in which it appears that the news media are doing their job.

A second strategy is to retreat into areas of representation so vague they cannot be contested by an appeal to facticity. There is no better example of this strategy than the creation of the "threat index" by the U.S. Government's Department of Homeland Security. This "threat index" is religiously reported by the news media whenever the government gives the call. The threat index allegedly lets the public know the level of imminence regarding a near future terrorist attack. The index does not tell where, when, or how such an event will occur, it merely says that an attack is less probable or more probable than in the near past. Moreover, its foundation is supposedly "credible evidence" gathered by an unknown—presumably government—agency and legitimized by an unknown source. Further, the indicators of what constitutes "credible evidence" have never been disclosed. Speculation has it that it can be anything from a "credible informant" to increased enemy chatter on the airwaves. All that is actually known is that Homeland Security says a real threat exists. Although the index is perpetually wrong as nothing has happened since its first appearance, it continues to be exchanged as an empty sign of threat—there to help the public stay prepared.

In situations such as this, biowarfare comes to be a great ally of those who benefit by the perpetuation of the representation of crisis. Mass body invasion by germs is always one of the potential threats to which the index may refer. This fearsome possibility can then be reinforced by the news fictionalists that are presented to the public as expert consultants. As if this is not enough, mass spectacles of under-preparedness are simulated in cities around the United States in conjunction with the federal government. Coverage of these media circuses circulates on the airwaves and in newspapers nationwide. Images of the fallen and of people in spooky decontamination suits spraying disinfectant create a greater spectacle of fear, which in turn engenders more discussion of apocalyptic scenarios. (We will return to this issue in the chapter on the spectacle of public health.) In all this media hype, never is the public reminded that an incident of germ warfare has happened only once, or that the origin of the germs used for that attack was the U.S. military. Rather, the public is only left with the fear that attacks could occur, along with a profound sense of disempowerment that reinforces the deferment of protective function to the state.

Should the news media refuse to see their interests as aligning with government policy and its need for the perpetuation of crisis, the state has punishment mechanisms at its disposal. Both the government (primarily the office of the president) and the military can deny access to media functions such as press conferences. One would think that this punishment would be a minor inconvenience, but here the state can exploit the news media's own warped priorities. The value of the media getting a story first has come to hold greater significance than quality reporting. Without access to presidential press functions, the individual news media companies fear they will lose viewers due to lack of speed; they will fall behind the discussion curve and fall into irrelevance for the viewer. As with so many institutions in the time of postmodernity, speed is a greater generator of profit than quality or integrity. What makes this situation even more absurd is that the differential between getting the scoop first and getting left in the dust is only a matter of minutes–and often even less than that. It's quite possible that getting the scoop first is a value that is only perceived by the press itself. If the separation between networks on getting a story is only a matter of minutes, who besides the most dedicated of channel surfers with multiple televisions would ever know the difference?

What the public gets in the end is a monstrous propaganda machine that functions as a finger on the thrusting fist of authority. The news media is one of many institutions that aids in the internalization of the hyperreality of crisis in general and the crisis in biointegrity in particular. A mode of consciousness is created in which the public comes to desire its state of fear and even feel protective of it. The delivery of contrary information—and thereby the denial of the immediacy of crisis—is often met with angry skepticism as if something of value is being taken from individuals. Leaving the security of hyperreality and the comfort of panic (both having established themselves in bodies, in desire, and in performativity) becomes a suicidal or murderous possibility, prompting a public demand for the consolidation and perpetuation of state violence.

Time to Get Paid

The APVs that benefit from the general situation of terror are making maximum gains. They are extracting more profit and consolidating more power than was probably ever expected. But the loss is not only limited to a redistribution of wealth and power in favor of the already abundantly wealthy and powerful; it goes on to extract life from those within the least powerful demographics. In terms of public policy regarding public health and global health, as we shall see in later chapters, the cost is a literal holocaust, as millions die worldwide every year of AIDS, malaria, cholera, tuberculosis, influenza, and dysentery. As people consume the hyperreality of bioterrorism, they miss the true crisis right in front of their eyes.

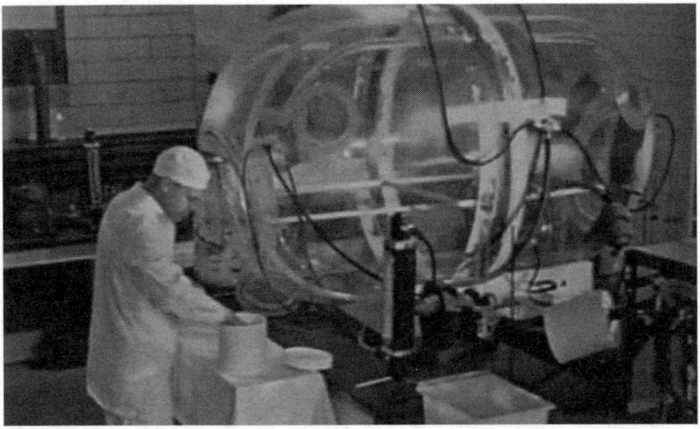

On September 4, 2001, the New York Times revealed that the United States had developed classified biodefense programs indistinguishable from offensive germ warfare research. Begun during the Clinton administration, the projects were expanded under Bush. The United States kept the projects secret and did not divulge them in annual reports to the Bioweapons Convention.

In one project, the CIA built and tested a cluster bomb that could spread biological agents over a wide area. The Pentagon's Threat Reduction Agency built a bioweapons plant from commercially available materials in the Nevada desert to demonstrate the alleged ease with which such a project could be undertaken by terrorists or rogue states without raising suspicions. The Defense Intelligence Agency tried to genetically engineer more powerful anthrax to replicate a Russian strain thought to be resistant to U.S. military vaccinations.

The United States maintains that these programs are defensive, claiming that in order to manufacture vaccines and develop defenses against biological attacks, researchers must first be able to produce the weapons.

3

Impossible Treaties

When scanning histories of failed progressive and radical causes, one cannot help but notice how nice it would be if more were actually successful—alternative fuels, an end to racism (or even just Jim Crow), free electricity, universal health care, a living minimum wage, and on and on. Right in line with this particular tradition of failure are treaties banning weapons of mass destruction and the use and production of weapons that cause undue suffering. The focus in this area has primarily been on chemical weapons. It is a history that began with a glimmer of hope.

The first international agreement limiting the use of chemical weapons dates back to 1675, when France and Germany came to an agreement signed in Strasbourg prohibiting the use of poison bullets. The treaty was limited, specific, and only between two countries. Simplicity tends to help, but this was the first and last of the successful treaties in the line leading to the Biological Weapons Convention (BWC, 1972/75).

The next attempt at curbing chemical warfare was 200 years later in 1874 at the Brussels Convention on the Laws and Customs of War. This convention was called by Tsar Alexander II and had a broad European attendance. A document was drafted that prohibited the use of poison or poisoned weapons (*On Hostilities*, Chapter 1, Article 23A) and the use of arms, projectiles or material to cause unnecessary suffering (23E). The document was not enthusiastically received, and a number of countries refused to sign. The timing of the convention is often deemed to have played a large part in its downfall. In the immediate aftermath of the Crimean War, the American Civil War, and the Franco-Prussian War, military and political delegates were quite reticent about agreeing to anything regarding arms limitations. The need for this treaty became all the more urgent as war technology "advanced" with the production of modern day chemical weapons. Before the turn of the century, a third attempt was made to obtain a consensus on the rules of war, and part of that discussion involved chemical weapons. An international peace conference was held in The Hague in 1899, at which delegates from twenty-six countries were present. These were Germany, the United States of America, Austria-Hungary, Belgium, China, Denmark, Spain, France, Great Britain and Ireland, Greece, Italy, Japan, Luxembourg, Mexico, Montenegro, the Netherlands, Persia, Portugal, Romania, Russia, Serbia, Siam, Sweden and Norway, Switzerland, Turkey, and Bulgaria. Among the documents produced, one prohibiting the use of projectiles filled with poison gas was advanced for signature. Only 15 countries signed the document.

The document was flawed from the beginning. Since it only prohibited the "use" of chemical weapons, the development of chemical warfare programs went unabated, and since not all delegates signed, countries reserved the right to chemically attack those countries that did not sign and to respond in kind to anyone that attacked them. The news only got worse. After the start of World War I, any signature on any treaty was quickly forgotten. All weapons were usable weapons. The carnage for both military and civilian personnel was horrific. Germany is generally credited with the first use of asphyxiating gases when it released chlorine gas in Ypres, Belgium in 1915, but there is plenty of blame to go around. As the war came to a close, provisions were introduced into the Treaty of Versailles that prohibited Germany, Bulgaria, Austria, and Hungary from using, manufacturing, or importing chemical weapons. These modest prohibitions were clearly not enough to stop a military performance such as World War I from being repeated. With the memories of chemical attacks still fresh, another convention was called in Geneva to try yet again to ban these weapons.

This convention produced a document that banned the use of asphyxiating, poisonous, or other gases as a method of warfare. The Polish delegation suggested that bacteriological methods of warfare also be banned. This was the beginning of an attempted ban on biological weapons. Again, the treaty was flawed since it did not prohibit the development, production, or possession of chemical weapons. It only banned the use of chemical and bacteriological (biological) weapons in war. Moreover, many countries signed the Protocol with reservations permitting them to use chemical weapons against countries that had not joined the treaty or to respond in kind if attacked with chemical weapons. But most damning is that a majority of countries neither signed when the treaty opened for signature in 1925, nor after it entered into force in 1928. Only France, Italy, Austria, Belgium, Liberia, and Russia signed the treaty before it went into effect in 1928. Germany held out until 1929, and Poland (the originator of the first anti-germ-warfare legislation) also signed in 1929. Most nations were serious latecomers, including the United States, which signed the protocol in 1975.

A final attempt to get the necessary treaty counterpart to the Geneva Convention protocols of 1925 occurred in 1971. The hope was to get the development, production, stockpiling, and acquisition of biological weapons linked to the use prohibitions of the Geneva agreement. (Chemical weapons had already been covered in other treaty initiatives.) This diplomatic push originated in the United States during the Nixon administration. Two important trends dovetailed (no pun intended) to allow what could only be viewed at the time as a surprise diplomatic move by the United States. Nixon had been told since the late 1960s that the germ warfare program was a bust and that little could be done with this form of weaponry. Nixon also knew that the Kennedy administration had received similar advice. Unfortunately for Kennedy, history was against him. After so much hype had gone into the importance of the germ warfare program, he felt he could not back away from it. To do so, he believed, would have infuriated the American public, as earlier research would have been seen as a tremendous waste of taxpayer dollars. Rather than saying a mistake had been made, Kennedy elected to continue with the program. By 1971, during the Nixon administration, the

American public was completely infuriated by military waste, so they responded positively to the treaty and the end of such a program once and for all. Moreover, Nixon got a double return. On one hand, he could begin to appease the popular peace movement, and he could begin reshaping his image as a war criminal into that of one who wants to stop war crimes—a smart move given the presidential election on the horizon.

The document that emerged from the 1971 meetings was the Convention on the Prohibition of the Development, Production, and Stockpiling of Bacteriological (Biological) and Toxin Weapons and on their Destruction (also referred to as the Biological Weapons Convention, BWC). The treaty opened for signatures in April 1972 (before the elections in the United States) and entered into force in 1975. This treaty does not prohibit use, but defers to the Geneva Convention and International Law on this matter. Its key prohibitions read as follows:

> *Each State Party to this Convention undertakes never in any circumstances to develop, produce, stockpile, or otherwise acquire or retain:*
>
> *1. Microbial or other biological agents, or toxins whatever their origin or method of production, of types and in quantities that have no justification for prophylactic, protective or other peaceful purpose;*
>
> *2. Weapons, equipment or means of delivery designed to use such agents or toxins for hostile purposes or in armed conflict.*

Over 100 countries have signed the treaty. Twenty-six nations have not. The only military power still refusing to sign is Israel.

This document sounds principled and practical, but in actuality it is not. The treaty itself has been an abysmal failure. Since 1972, the number of germ warfare programs has consistently grown. More programs exist now than ever before. The United States is substantially expanding its germ warfare program. What was a minor military program in the 1970s has now returned to its glory days of the 1950s and 1960s.

Offense Is Defense

While there are many factors that land the BWC in the realm of hopelessness, no greater reason exists than the clause in the treaty that allows for defensive germ warfare programs. This escape hatch of a clause essentially makes any program legal and legitimate, since separating the defensive from the offensive is nearly impossible. Only two sectors of a given program are affected. The first is stockpiling. A justification for collecting massive amounts of bioweaponry has yet to be devised. The second sector is mass production. A nation does not need to have the facilities to mass-produce germs. So a small nod to the elimination of biological weapons could potentially be given by signatory countries. In the United States, where the germ warfare program is expanding at an alarming rate, at least the germ manufacturing facility at Fort Detrick was dismantled. If this was the only facility, it would indicate that mass manufacture and stockpiling have probably also stopped. Unfortunately, due to the absence of verification protocols, no one will ever know for sure.

But here is the really bad news: every other element of the germ warfare program is still on the table. That means new transgenic germs that could be weaponized are being produced, along with new delivery systems, new detection systems, and vaccine development. Moreover, germs that should no longer exist anywhere on earth are being preserved. All of these program elements are defensive, but they are at one and the same time necessary components for offensive weapons programs. The way this scam works is very simple. All that is required for an element of a germ warfare program to be deemed defensive is a plausible reason that it is. The fact that the element can also serve in an offensive situation is then ignored. One might ask, how can a delivery system be a defensive weapon? As the logic goes, if the system is not linked to stockpiling, then the nation is simply looking into delivery possibilities in order to be able to protect its citizens should that delivery system ever be used. This is precisely why germ warfare programs are expanding under this well-intentioned but useless treaty. The logic is so twisted that it could make heads explode. A technology exists only as a paranoid fantasy, but then it is designed and manufactured so that the public can be protected from it. The bizarre notion that the need to neutralize a threat predates the threat itself is simply insane. And, expanding the range of possibility of threat in order to manufacture a better form of security makes even less sense. The "defense" industry has found a way to expand itself in perpetuity. As long as the military can continuously imagine additional threatening possibilities, it can keep making nightmares into realities for its own benefit.

What is additionally sinister is that the only people that tend to die from germ warfare programs are the citizens of the nation that program is supposedly protecting. History has shown this over and over. The Russians never killed anyone with their advanced and immense germ warfare program with the exception of those Russian citizens killed at Sverdlovsk during a tragic anthrax accident. The only people killed by the United States program were Americans. Two workers associated with the program died of anthrax exposure—one in 1951 and another in 1958. Another one died in 1964 of Bolivian hemorrhagic fever. In 1968, in the final year of the program, a janitor died when he was exposed to anthrax while changing a light bulb. These are only the deaths that the military will admit happened. The deaths of five people in 2001 of anthrax exposure are a little more mysterious. In all probability the anthrax was created by and belonged to the U.S. germ warfare program. At the very least, the U.S. military's recipe for creating weapons grade germs was used by those who produced the anthrax. Since army personnel were the only ones with access to it, let speculation fall where it may. Moreover, during the period between 1942 and 1969 (the good ol' days of germ warfare), 419 personnel became ill with various diseases. When the program was reduced in the 1970s and 1980s, only five people associated with the program became ill. Expansion of a program does not lead to security, but precisely to the very opposite: an enhanced probability that an accident will happen or that someone will find a little on-the-side testing to be an irresistible attractor.

New germs or delivery systems are clearly dual-natured in terms of military capability, but what about the more innocuous elements? How could a detection system be a part of an offensive program? To be sure, a detection system is an integral part of a defensive safety shield. The ability to identify the appearance of contamination, its type, projected rate, and/or area of coverage is a necessity for a quick and effective response. (The questions here are who should create detection equipment, who will prioritize the need for different detectors that are sensitive to different germs, and who should respond if contamination has occurred. These will be discussed in later chapters.) Be that as it may, this technology has offensive capabilities, since a military would want to verify that it has effectively contaminated enemy territory and then track the contamination so as to avoid blowback. Any element of a defensive program is reversible, which is the primary reason the BWC is so ineffective.

Another example is vaccines. How could vaccines be anything but benign? Vaccines may be benign, but what are they protecting us from? The emergence of transgenics has all but made vaccines an anachronism. Once a vaccine is developed, a germ can be genetically restructured to be resistant to the vaccine. As with delivery systems, this formula can be reversed. First, the germs are manufactured, then the vaccine is manufactured to neutralize them. This cycle can go on into infinitude. Through this method, a germ warfare program can expand in quality if not in quantity. While there may not be stockpiles, there will be a massive, ever growing library of new organisms capable of killing humans and the organic matter that supports human life (crops, for example).

As CAE has stated in previous chapters, but which always bears repeating: the only terrorists that are going to use biological weapons against the United States are its own military branches. Even the military's Office of Technological Assessment has said that it is extremely improbable that terrorists would use such weaponry (even if they could get it, transport it, and deploy it to begin with). The reasons they give are lack of familiarity, fear of alienating supporters by causing large numbers of casualties, fear of an extreme response by another country, fear of working with biological weapons, prohibition by terrorist groups' financial sponsors, and the need to await someone else's successful use. Some of these reasons are contradictory, but all are possible and plausible. Terrorists are not deranged humans looking to spread chaos as if they were the Legion of Doom or some other comic book fabrication. They have a political agenda; they are strategically as well as tactically goal-oriented; and thereby have limits placed upon them by what they desire to achieve.

The Big Flip Flop

Back in the glory days of the American germ warfare program, the idea that offensive and defensive weapons and support systems were inseparable was common wisdom. Since no threat to research budgets existed, the military was willing to call it like it saw it. As the Office of the Secretary of Defense said in 1949 (when it was just beginning to push the idea of germ warfare and needed to show what good value it was): "Information obtained from research on the defensive aspect of BW [biological warfare] is, in the greater part, applicable to offensive weapons as well." The government was all set for a military two-fer. The commitment to this way of thinking about BW never wavered throughout the glory days. In 1968, the final year of carte blanche, the army still maintained that what was good for offense was good for the defense. As this quote from Richard Clendenin, a historian from the Technical Information Division at Fort Detrick indicates: "...research and development in the offensive aspect of BW proceeded hand in hand with defensive developments for, in truth, the two are almost inseparable." Here we have a military historian chronicling how the program had proceeded over the past twenty plus years. During that time, it was a given that offense and defense were inseparable.

In 1969 it became clear that the germ warfare program was about to be seriously cut. By 1971, offensive weapons were being taken off the table, not just by the Nixon administration, but also by international law. It was then that the U.S. military reversed its position. All of a sudden, offense and defense had nothing to do with each other. This position has been maintained to this day and is now the newspeak of common BW wisdom. While the original position of "two for one" value may have been exaggerated in order to make the initial sale, it was at least in the realm of the real. The new position by the military and White House administrations since Reagan is so disingenuous that it sounds worse than fingernails scraping across a blackboard. While it is true that offensive and defensive research are not exactly the same, the similarities far outweigh the differences.

Verification

The second major problem with the BWC treaty is that it has no verification protocols. None. If a signature nation is cheating, there is no way to verify this as long as the cheats are competent. While there was discussion of verification protocols from the beginning, it never went far. The discussions never even seriously began until the early 1990s. Throughout this period and into the present, the United States, it seems, has preferred that verification does not occur. In fact, Bush went so far as to sabotage the 2001 meetings during which a consensus on verification seemed to be on the verge of actuation. Bush pulled out of the verification agreement with the explanation that the protocols would have a negative impact on U.S. commercial interests. This is not unusual: the United States has met very few treaties on arms limitations of which it has approved—even those it has sponsored, as in this case. The United States still has not ratified the treaty to eliminate incendiary bombs. Other nations should not get between the U.S. military and its napalm.

While Bush's explanation was primarily disingenuous, a grain of truth can be found. What creates this sticking point is the method by which verification is done. The example of the Iraq weapons inspection is quite telling as to why the United States would prefer not to have these inspections. The Iraq inspections, as all others would, took a very long time. When the inspection team was recalled months after they had started, the inspections were still not complete. Inspections are not simply a matter of entering a suspicious factory and having Mr. Spock take a tricorder reading. Tests have to occur repeatedly at numerous sites in conjunction with constant cross-referencing of all evidence gathered. The method is one of slow investigation in which the same piece of evidence that indicates a violation may just as easily indicate innocence. During the Iraq inspection, media audiences were constantly being told that traces of chemical weapons were being found. The Iraqis said it was insecticide. Either explanation could have been true. What was eventually discovered by military experience in Iraq (and by U.N. weapons inspectors who were summarily ignored by the Bush Administration) was that it probably *was* only insecticide. In inspections, clues have to be linked to an extent that an emergent, holistic picture of the situation comes to light. Until that tipping point is reached, the evidence represents little more than a minor possibility.

From the perspective of the Bush administration, international inspectors wandering through corporate and military installations' most sensitive areas serve only to invite enemy corporate and military espionage. This scenario is plausible, but unlikely. However, since it is plausible, both military and corporate entities would rather not take any chances. Pharmaceutical companies involved in transgenic and vaccine research have complained quite bitterly that their trade secrets could be compromised. Certainly, the vast sums of money given to the Republican Party and the strength of the pharmaceutical lobby have had some effect on Bush's decision to withdraw from verification procedures. The lesson here is that authoritarian power vectors would rather not increase global security with regard to WMDs if accomplishing this goal comes at the expense of corporate profits.

What if a presidential administration actually cared for people more than profits, and accepted the verification protocols? Hell would be freezing over, but in addition to that, a problem with the BWC would still continue. What could be done if someone was caught cheating? In fact, this has happened. Returning to the disaster at Sverdlovsk, one can, with reasonable assurance, say that the Russians had overstepped the limits of the treaty. If a factory manufacturing anthrax has a malfunction that causes military grade anthrax to be sprayed over four square kilometers, it seems fair to say that an offensive BW program exists. The United States said just this, but what could be done? A "justified" war with Russia was a possibility, but happily, that was rejected. Those were the only options on the table beyond making a diplomatic fuss.

There is Never a Cop Around When You Need One

If atrocity-for-atrocity politics are to be avoided, or at least undermined, can a peaceful alternative be found? Noam Chomsky's vision of restraint in conjunction with following procedures and processes of international law as a means to avoid illegal military program expansion is seductive. The process of investigation and presentation of evidence, along with the pursuit of a global consensus concerning guilt, certainly sounds much better than the current "for us or against us" model employed by the United States and Britain. Theoretically, Islamic nations would be included in this process in a manner that would not appear to their respective citizens as an obsequious charade forced by Western economic and/or military pressure. Such a process would, of course, start with a treaty like the BWC.

While the goals of this alternative appear healthy and desirable, the problems of implementation are such that it borders on being naive. CAE will refrain from discussing all of the problems in this section and will instead focus on a singular key issue–the structure of international law and treaty enforcement by the World Court. Lessons have been learned about the function of these institutions from the experience of less powerful nations trying to be good global citizens. One clear example is Nicaragua. During the United States' "illegal" (under international law) military, economic, and ideological assault on this nation in the 1980s, Nicaragua attempted to defend itself against this superpower by appealing to the World Court. This august body actually ruled in favor of Nicaragua, ordering the United States to cease hostilities and pay reparations. The United States ignored the judgment. Nicaragua then went to the United Nations Security Council, only to have the United States veto a resolution that called for nations to observe international law.

What does this tell us about the current crisis regarding BW, given that the situation is inverted? After all, we are not witnessing a powerless nation demanding justice from a powerful one; rather, a superpower is being asked to follow international law in the face of what it perceives as an act of war against which it must defend itself. The answer is the same as with the Nicaraguan example: a superpower is not compelled to follow law; it creates, modifies, or ignores the law to suit its interests. International law and the World Court are, in the grand majority of cases, tools of capital (and of U.S. capital in particular) designed to paint a just face upon its activities. More to the point, laws and courts are only as powerful as their ability to enforce their decisions. To accomplish the task of dispensing justice, they must be intimately linked to a complex repressive apparatus primarily consisting of the Virilio twins: vision (surveillance systems) and violence (a policing body in charge of enforcement and containment).

The relationship of the World Court to a policing body is simple to describe: The U.S. military is its police force. Hence, when the court acts in the interest of capital, it is a powerful judicial institution because its verdicts and penalties are enforced; when the court acts contrary to capital, it is a woefully impotent institution. As for the Iraq crisis, the Bush administration appears to believe that the U.S. military is doing its work quite capably, so why chance potential legal restrictions that could disrupt its "just" enforcement procedures? Even if the United States were to go through the legal process before acting, how would the outcome be any different, other than that military action would be slightly delayed, and a greater spectacle of justice would potentially polish the surface of the corrupt initiative? Going to the World Court is either only a symbolic gesture void of material results (Nicaragua) or an indirect appeal for U.S. military (police) action, as opposed to an alternative to it. The United States does need not to ask itself for permission to deploy its military might. (CAE should note that the World Court also functions as an arbiter of punishment for enemies of capital that have already been militarily dispatched, such as Slobodan Milosevic). As long as international law is dependent on superpower enforcement, there will never be a cop around when you need one.

In spite of the fact that the BWC has caused the expansion of germ warfare programs, has no verification protocols, has no possibility of enforcement, and still allows for defensive weapons that are indistinguishable from offensive ones, one good thing can be said about it: it reinforces the idea that the use and manufacture of these weapons is unacceptable in the eyes of the global community. Regardless of the material disaster that this treaty has failed to stop, it does offer an exchangeable sign in the marketplace of ideas that helps to maintain the feelings of personal repulsion and the thoughts of global suicide that are associated with this type of weaponry. While even this potentially positive element is exploited by militaries and governments to manufacture fear, it may also be the best defense thus far for maintaining a germ-free peace.

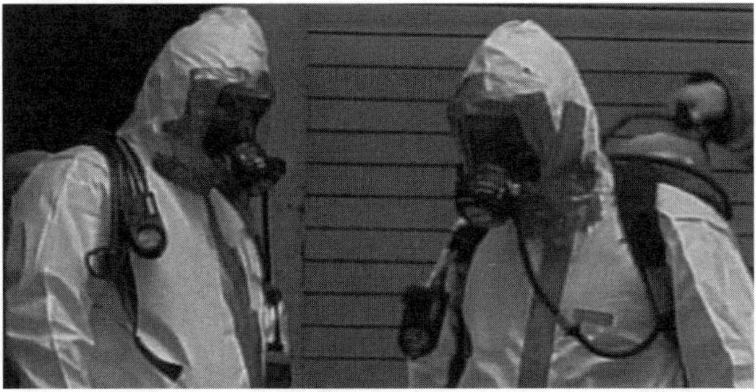

What makes a nanocomposite material "smart"? Consider clothing that can detect the presence of chemical weapons, automatically seal its own pores, and then clean and decontaminate itself. Today the U.S. Department of Defense is funding research for fabric materials that do all these things and are also stronger, more durable, and lighter than current uniforms.

Smart materials are becoming a reality, and one of the world's leading experts in the field is Sergiy Minko, who holds the Egon Matijevic Chair of Chemistry at Clarkson University.

One of Minko's current projects involves research into self-cleaning fabrics sponsored by the National Textile Center. Made of any common fabric, these materials will utilize a water-repellant, dirt-repellant, environment-friendly coating made of silver nanoparticles. Their wide applications will include hospital and military garments, as well as sportswear, awnings, and convertible tops.

4

The Spectacle of Public Health Under the Sign of Bioterror

When examining the tendencies of capitalism, its praise for and application of the principles of efficiency, utility, and functionality often dominate analysis. Even when considering the oppressive mechanisms of capitalist power vectors, the critical use of the three principles has considerable explanatory power. Yet areas exist where these principles tend to obscure elements of specific varieties of system failure. For over ten years, CAE has been arguing that the nonrational principles of waste, uselessness, and human sacrifice can be of particular explanatory value where capital's own self description, due to its inherent contradictions, fails to produce a sufficient or accurate overview.

The capitalist tendencies toward waste, uselessness, and sacrifice serve a dual purpose. On the one hand, they must be acknowledged as existing in noncapitalist social systems. Yet they must be hidden within capitalism itself, so that their absence can act as an alibi for the productive principles that the bureaucratic and technocratic strata of capitalism so dearly embrace. The apparent absence of uselessness demonstrates that production is always useful; the absence of waste demonstrates that resources are universally linked to efficiency; and the absence of sacrifice demonstrates that the system is just. On the other hand, a firm connection to these nonrational material relationships by dynamic forces of domination is the ultimate expression of raw power. Who but the most powerful can waste life and resources on pointless endeavors without regard for utility or profit? A quasi-controlled participation in such activity is the greatest reward within capitalism, and yet no individual or group can remain master of the under-economy (the sphere of the social nonrational) for an extended period. The realm of the nonrational is in a constant process of deterritorialization and will destroy that which attempts to stifle the process.

In the discourse on public health, these principles of the under-economy are of tremendous explanatory value. The current spectacle of security through militarized public health initiatives intersects all the worst tendencies of the under-economy. Capital has perverted the redeeming power of the nonrational by stripping away anything positive that could emerge from it and leaving only its authoritarian possibilities. In the case of public health, fighting disease and intensifying public preparedness for real, ongoing health crises is no longer a valued, humanitarian initiative; instead, we have a military flight of fantasy that prioritizes the fantastic and improbable over the real and certain. This unfortunate state of affairs actually puts the public in greater danger of medical disaster from any type of pandemic and wastes billions of dollars on useless equipment, vaccines, and emergency planning for highly improbable events such as biowarfare, while ignoring the disasters that are actually happening, such as multi-drug resistant tuberculosis or hepatitis C, which are not of military value (i.e., not useful in warfare).

Waste and Excess

In their fundamental forms, societies were protected from the emergence of capitalism by their relationship to waste. By disallowing the centralization and consolidation of the means to power, simple societies (i.e., those with a modest division of labor) minimized the opportunity for huge separations and inequalities to develop. One common material manifestation of this collective desire is the potlatch. Here an individual would collect personal property until it reached the crisis point of becoming private property; that is, until so much had been collected that it could no longer be used by the individual. At this point, the excess property would begin to generate the need for a market and the opportunity to make profit. Rather than taking this fatal step, the property would be redistributed by the owner to the other members of the society in one generous, yet often wasteful, gesture.

In contrast, capitalism is dependent on market creation and expansion, and embraces the separations that accompany a complex division of labor. Within this political-economic configuration, capital would have people believe that waste has been eliminated. To be sure, waste is not good for minimizing consumer prices, and those competing for market share can little afford to treat their resources in a cavalier way. Producers' survival in the marketplace is dependent upon their efficiency in relation to other producers competing for the same slice of the market. Due to such imperatives, the capitalist political economy has emerged as the wealthiest, most complex, and most technologically advanced society in history. The evidence is overwhelming that this position is accurate, yet an ideological sleight of hand is occurring. As profit accumulates, it can't all return as reinvestment. Some must be spent in other ways, and this spending is where capital forges one of its links to waste. A vast amount of profit and wages (in the form of taxes) must be spent on maintaining and protecting the sphere of production itself. The jewel in the crown of capitalist waste is its standing army. An unused military produces nothing and eats resources and profit at an astounding rate. Even when used, it still runs at a huge deficit. The primary function of the army is to gorge itself on as much profit and wages as it can in order to become an even larger, hungrier monster.

The second relation to waste is spending on spectacles and simulations designed to convince people that something that does not exist actually does. These are not the spectacles of late imperial Rome in which lavish sums of public monies were wasted on plebian entertainment; rather, these spectacles and simulations function to glorify authoritarian imaginaries that will never materially manifest. The current mythology of terrorists acquiring weapons of mass destruction and destroying the United States "in a mushroom cloud"—a key talking point in the build up to the Iraq war—is patently absurd. ("Weapons of mass distraction" was certainly a point of sloganeering truth.) Very few countries have the capacity to produce nuclear weapons, but why would those that do give them to terrorists? If a nation has gone to the trouble of acquiring these weapons, it would be political insanity to give the most important weapon in its arsenal to a group whose intentions are unknown. Why give the best weapon to someone who could one day be an enemy? Certainly the case of the U.S. support of "freedom fighters" (now terrorists) in Afghanistan is but one lesson learned. "Conventional arms only" is the order of the day when it comes to supplying independent military organizations.

The point where the real amusement begins is when power vectors get caught in their own iron cage of spectacle and have no choice but to comply with the demands of the spectacle. The United States is stuck with an expanding germ warfare program in part because so much was made of the threatening specter of bioterrorism. Moreover, terrible logistical blunders in Iraq were made because of the fantasy concerning Iraqi use of chemical and biological weapons. While U.S. soldiers have all had anthrax vaccines and have full protective gear for such attacks (that have never happened), they lack proper armor for their vehicles, adequate body armor, and a sufficient number of armored transport vehicles. The priorities of equipping the army have become completely skewed. Equipping soldiers for a remote possibility is more important than equipping them for the small arms fire occurring on a daily basis. Indeed, this distortion of the real and the actions that have followed are parallel to issues of global public health, in which the diseases that kill masses of people every day are considered less important than diseases that have only rarely killed anyone.

Uselessness

Of all the principles most abhorrent to capitalist society, uselessness must rank near the top. It could be the most repulsive quality relative to capitalist values. Uselessness is generally a disciplinary term used to label people who refuse to participate in the system. Dropouts, drug addicts, welfare recipients, and the lumpenproletariat (the "dangerous classes") in general are all candidates for the reprimand of uselessness. However, while uselessness may contradict capitalist ideological imperatives, examples of it are everywhere and intersect heavily with waste.

Uselessness is far more interesting when it is analyzed not as a visible, disciplinary label, but rather, as a hidden property that haunts the world of the functional. We find uselessness even in the most functional of items, such as simple and complex technologies. Technology is generally considered a practical, material formation. Sometimes its tendency is utopian, sometimes apocalyptic, but it is always assumed to be functioning instrumentally. In truth, instrumentality's opposition very often creeps into the techno-object. From low-end instruments like cell phones jammed with useless features (where many of the more esoteric features are really there as ends in themselves), to the many overly specialized pieces of low-end technology that clutter the closets of the middle class, to the highest-end germ and nuclear warfare technologies, uselessness is an integral part of each. When has the intercontinental ballistic missile ever been used? The technology is assembled only to be disassembled and removed to make way for the next generation of useless war-tech. As with the logic of germ warfare program expansion, the logic of this system can make minds melt. Should this technology ever function, it has failed to serve a purpose. Given this non-functional purpose, the intercontinental system does not even have to work at all; it must only succeed in appearing to work.

The same may be said about germ warfare. If it doesn't remain useless it has failed its purpose, but the fantasy of its use must be acknowledged as real as often as possible. The appearance of functionality is important, and considerable resources are pumped into the hype surrounding this technology. As we have documented in past chapters, biological weapons are completely unpredictable and unreliable, but the facts do not matter. As we have shown in chapter two, there is too much money at stake. Only the fantasy is relevant. Without the fantasy, biological weapons are only what they are—useless junk.

Other elements of the germ warfare program share these same qualities of uselessness and waste, including those that are supposed to support public health. The center of this massive waste of revenue is the vaccine initiative sponsored by the National Institute of Allergy and Infectious Disease (NIAID). How could a vaccination program be a problem? Citizens may not get a good return on their investment, but at least the program can't hurt anything, and it may in fact help. While this logic sounds convincing, the facts suggest otherwise.

First, we must begin with the question of the two top concerns in regard to germ warfare: anthrax and smallpox. Second, we must ask whether there is any imminent threat from these germs. The NIAID will begrudgingly admit, "At present, there is no specific information to indicate that there is a likelihood of use of anthrax or smallpox as a weapon in the immediate future." When asked what the consequences are should such a weapon be used, the response is, "While we cannot quantify the threat of either one being used as a bioweapon, we know the consequences of their use would be great." While it sounds as if a certain clear and present danger exists, what this statement actually means when viewed through the lens of scientific rigor is that NIAID officials have no idea what the destructive capability is, but their guess is that it could be bad. This spectacle of crisis and catastrophe is a fantasy, but one that must be engaged immediately. What is the reward for accepting fantasy as reality? The U.S. government is funding three new biosafety level four labs (built for research on the most infectious and virulent germs): one at Rocky Mountain Laboratories in Hamilton, Montana at a cost of 66.5 million dollars, one at Fort Detrick, Maryland (the center of germ warfare research) at a cost of 105 million dollars, and of course, Building 33 on the National Institutes of Health's campus at a cost of 186.1 million dollars. Nine regional Biocontainment Laboratories with biosafety level three facilities are in planning or under construction. This initiative was slow since some local residents were not keen on having these labs in their neighborhoods. Here are some of the germs to be studied in the BSL3 labs:

Anthrax
Respiratory viral pathogens
Poxviruses (e.g., Vaccinia)
Tuberculosis
Tularemia
Enteric pathogens
Vector-borne flaviviruses, including West Nile virus

One has to wonder if this is what is in a BSL3, what is being studied in the BSL4 labs? Be that as it may, the payoff for supporting the fantasy is big. But there is more. In order to better militarize academia, the NIAID has funded ten Regional Centers of Excellence (RCE) for Biodefense and Emerging Infectious Disease Research. RCE grants have been awarded to Harvard Medical School, Duke University, the University of Chicago, the University of Maryland, the University of Texas Medical Branch, the University of Washington, and Washington University. (Other locations have not been confirmed.) At first glance, this effort also sounds good, but what it really means is that the centers' primary concern will be military interests rather than those pertaining to public health, and it is these concerns that will direct infectious disease research. As we shall see, the two sets of priorities are far from similar.

The military and NIAID know what to say when asked about what they will study. A representative list on their website looks like this: "Plague, Lyme disease, rabies, tick-borne encephalitis, West Nile virus disease, influenza, anthrax infection, Ebola virus hemorrhagic fever, HIV, tuberculosis, transmissible spongiform encephalopathies, and Q fever." A number of these are diseases that have an immediate impact on public health, such as HIV, influenza, and tuberculosis. Perhaps CAE is incorrect, and the military is acting in the public interest rather than its own; however, once one examines the central initiatives where "progress" is being made, a different scenario develops.

Of greatest concern is smallpox. To begin with, natural cases of smallpox have been eradicated from the earth. The last natural case was recorded in 1977 in Somalia. The only reason it still exists and could be reintroduced into the environment at all is due to BW programs that are keeping it alive. In fact, the last case reported occurred in 1978 in Birmingham, England.

Improper lab procedures resulted in the death of Janet Parker. Ms. Parker was a medical photographer who worked in a lab above the one researching smallpox at the University of Birmingham. Authorities believe that the virus traveled in air currents up a service duct to the room where she worked. The scientist responsible killed himself shortly after her death.

Smallpox does make great spectacle, since this very ugly disease has such a gruesome past. Smallpox has probably killed more people than any other disease in history. Unfortunately for the military, it is not an effective weapon. Viruses cannot live without a host and have been dismal failures as weapons because of this trait. The smallpox virus is heat sensitive and dies as it dries. Moreover, the living conditions of most developed nations are not conducive to its spread. Smallpox requires prolonged face-to-face contact to spread efficiently. An outbreak these days would probably spread slowly in developed nations, and public health officials have considerable experience in controlling outbreaks. Regardless, everyone should be relieved to know that if this extremely unlikely emergency were ever to occur, NIAID has spent millions of dollars on a vaccine to cover everyone in the United States (300 million doses). If that is not enough, a new smallpox vaccine is in the works. The "classic" one eradicated the disease, but the new one offers less chance of extremely rare complications. With this vaccine, the NIAID may save as many as a handful of people that could not be saved otherwise.

The NIAID's second primary concern is anthrax. Anthrax can be successfully weaponized. In its spore form, it can even be placed in shells and bombs. As CAE has pointed out in previous chapters, anthrax, like all BWs, has had a very disappointing track record. But is it a public health hazard? The United States has reported 236 cases of anthrax between 1955 and 1999. Anthrax is really not a disease of intense urgency—although workers who labor with animal carcasses and products might be pleased, since they have the highest occupational chance of contracting anthrax. Regardless of this low intensity public threat, the NIAID is focusing on bringing a new vaccine to market. The old one works, but the new one requires fewer doses to reach immunity. Knowing that our soldiers and first responders will have fewer pricks in their arms should make us feel more secure. Vaxgen, Inc., the company contracted to produce the 75 million doses of the vaccine, is probably significantly more financially secure as well. How public health is actually improved by all this hoopla remains to be seen.

The NIAID goes on to say that anthrax is a "Category A" agent. These agents are considered the highest threat to national security due to their "ease of transmission, high rate of death or serious illness, and potential for causing panic." This list of priority qualities is odd to say the least. First, what is meant by "transmission?" Anthrax cannot be transmitted from person to person—no record of this happening exists anywhere. Maybe the NIAID authors meant something else, but it sure sounds as though they mean transmission from person to person. Second, what are the criteria for "the potential to cause panic?" How was this studied? During the October 2001 anthrax attack, CAE does not recall anyone panicking. The postal workers left the contaminated buildings in which they worked, got tested, and when the sites were cleaned up, they went back to work. The closest the population came to panic stemmed from the panic of the Department of Homeland Security, which rather than be seen doing nothing, told citizens to stay at home and seal their windows with plastic and duct tape.

The next priority is CAE's personal favorite, the ebola virus. Like anthrax and smallpox, it is also a Category A agent. Is it a public health risk? Until recently, only a few outbreaks of ebola hemorrhagic fever striking humans had been reported. The first two outbreaks were in 1976: one in Zaire and one in western Sudan. These were relatively large outbreaks, resulting in more than 550 cases and 340 deaths. A third outbreak, in 1979 in Sudan, was smaller, with 34 cases and 22 fatalities. More recently, outbreaks have occurred again in Zaire in 1995 and 1996, with 352 cases and 276 deaths, and in Gabon in 1996, with 60 cases and 45 deaths. The death toll is 683 from five outbreaks in Africa in recent history. It's hard to see this as an urgent public health risk next to HIV or tuberculosis (which together are annihilating entire communities in Africa and the rest of the world). For these diseases, 683 deaths is a typical hour. While millions will continue to die every year of HIV and TB, our germ warfare program has spent millions of healthcare dollars making an ebola vaccine.

Consider some of the other products of the germ warfare program:

Safe and effective alternatives to toxoid vaccine
Monoclonal antibodies
Polyclonal antibodies
Second generation anthrax vaccines (e.g., rPA)
Marburg hemorrhagic fever vaccines
Tularemia vaccines
Plague vaccines
Rift Valley Fever vaccines
Cell culture (e.g., Vero cell) based vaccines for influenza
Antivirals for smallpox and viral hemorrhagic fevers

With the exception of influenza (Category C), the listed germs are Category A agents. This product list suggests that Category A is the highest priority. Unfortunately, while the A-list germs may awaken scary fantasies in the minds of the military, they are not public health dangers. These two elements—military priority and public health priority—are almost completely unrelated.

CAE must also inquire how these categories are even created. The reasoning suggested above (ease of transmission, high rate of serious illness or death, or potential for causing panic) cannot be true. For example, why is smallpox a Category A and multi-drug resistant tuberculosis (MDTB) a Category C? MDTB is equally contagious; it has a similar mortality rate; unlike smallpox, it's incredibly difficult to treat (which is in part responsible for its high mortality rate); it's an astronomically bigger drain on medical resources; and, unlike smallpox, it is already killing people in New York, California, and Texas. TB itself is the most infectious disease globally, infecting nearly one third of the world's population and killing two to three million people every year. The only possible argument that could be made on behalf of smallpox is that it would cause panic, while MDTB is already in the United States population and has not caused panic. This position is as arbitrary as the categories. Ultimately, the military is more obsessed with its fantasy about smallpox than the reality of TB.

Other diseases that make the A list also have no relation to public health crises and register as significant only because the military is interested in them for one paranoid reason or another. Tularemia, also known as "rabbit fever," is not even a blip on the public health radar. Approximately 200 cases of tularemia are reported each year. Less than two percent are fatal. Tularemia cannot be transmitted person to person, it is not highly infectious, and it doesn't seem to be causing panic. In the mind of the military, a big panic is underway. Tularemia is a bacteria, so it can live independently from a host. The germ is very versatile—it can be airborne, it can live in water, and it can live in mammals. It could be sprayed and inhaled, or it could be used to poison the food or water supply. Its one disadvantage is that it cannot take a spore form, so it cannot be placed in bombs. Tularemia is on the list not because it fits the Category A description, or causes panic in the general population, but because it makes the military panic.

Plague is on the A list, because it is really scary. From Thucydides' description of bubonic plague to the current military's fear that bioterrorists will use pneumonic plague (which, unlike bubonic plague, can be transmitted person to person), this virus has always been the King of the Fear Factor. It is gruesome, and it is contagious. Yet despite its regular appearance in the southwest United States (approximately 10 cases per year) it hasn't caused panic. The total number of cases on medical record worldwide amounts to 2,118. Moreover, plague is not a very good weapon. It is very sensitive to light and heat, and once deployed, under the best conditions, it can only live up to an hour without finding a host. From the time of the Japanese plague trials, to the British trials, to the United States trials, no military has been able successfully to use it tactically. In addition, it is treatable with antibiotics that already exist. However, millions more tax dollars are being spent to develop vaccines and more antibiotics to fight plague. As long as the military stays infatuated with the spectacle of a given disease, that disease is going to stay on the top-ten list and continue to consume resources that could be better used to save lives now.

One last note is necessary before leaving the realm of the useless and the wasteful, and that is in regard to stockpiling vaccines. Vaccines don't last. Most have to be replaced every six months to a year. Just like the missiles standing dumb in their silos waiting to be disassembled and replaced, so are the stores of vaccines. The logic of vaccine stockpiling is that if a nation has vaccines and in-kind retaliatory capability, it will deter an enemy from using biological weapons. Memories of Dr. Strangelove and the Russian doomsday machine come flooding back. Strangelove famously remarked that for a weapon to deter, everyone must know that a nation is in possession of it. As the United States publicly acknowledges the types of vaccines it has stockpiled, it allows the enemy the options of transgenically modifying the germ to thwart the vaccine, or simply using a bug for which the United States is unprepared. If the United States decides to keep their stockpiles a secret, they do not get the deterrence dividend. In the age of transgenics, stockpiling vaccines is little more than a very expensive publicity stunt offered to reinforce the public perception of security. Once again, the government and military offer empty spectacle to counter a perceived threat in order to look like they are doing something. The amount of resources wasted on useless material like stockpiles of vaccines is inexcusable, especially as it comes at the expense of people dying here and now from actual public health emergencies. Those who die are the sacrificial victims of the demented strategies of capital.

Human Sacrifice

Human sacrifice is typically assumed to be a "primitive" institution—one that long ago vanished from Western civilization. Unfortunately, quite the opposite is true. The institution of sacrifice lives on. Although much of it is hidden from view, it remains an essential part of first world everyday life, politics, and economy.*

Health care has long been among the primary sites of sacrifice in the United States. The thousands of deadly hospital mishaps and mistakes that occur each year are one of the unfortunate byproducts that citizens are willing to tolerate in order to have hospitals at all. While precautions are taken, people understand that perfect safety is not achievable and that a number of people must be sacrificed to this institution every year. To be sure, society always hopes to lower the number each year, but with an expanding system and an aging population more sacrifices will be required. The toleration of these deaths on an annual basis demonstrates that the population is sincere about the value and importance of having hospitals. This form of sacrifice is understandable, and to some degree unavoidable, much like the United States population must be willing to sacrifice approximately 40,000 people each year to continue automotive transportation.

---

*For a more complete discussion of human sacrifice in capitalist economy, please see Chapter 5 in *Electronic Civil Disobedience* (ECD). For a more complete discussion of useless technology, please see Chapter 4 in that same book.

However, truly pathological forms of human sacrifice also regularly occur in health care in the United States. The worst is due to the fact that the United States insists on being the only developed nation without universal heath care. The United States has the highest infant mortality rate in the developed world. Those in power are willing to sacrifice thousands of children each year to show they are sincere about the value of privatization and free market capitalism. To give mothers universal prenatal care or to ensure that all children are vaccinated would be tantamount to communism. While a commercial smallpox vaccination will be available to everyone who needs it, power vectors believe that a comprehensive vaccination program for children is going too far with the government handouts.

The relationship of authoritarian power vectors to emerging infectious disease is another point of pathological sacrifice. Given APVs' propensity for violence, emerging infectious disease is viewed primarily as a resource for violence. Those diseases that best fit military need to produce artificial forms of death are the ones focused upon, at the expense of diseases that are causing the catastrophic and present forms of natural death. The military has managed to reframe microbiology and health policy as arenas in which the improbable rules the actual. The cost is sacrifice. Millions must die to show sincerity and commitment to the "War on Terror." But the death of soldiers is not enough. As this chapter has shown, a sacrifice of the sick on a worldwide basis is yet more tribute that must be paid.

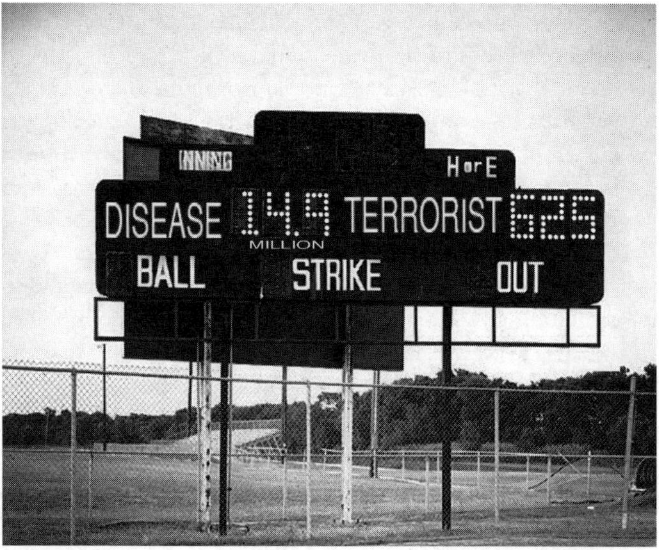

625 people died worldwide in 2003 from conventional terrorist attacks. There were no biological attacks reported. 14.9 million people died in 2002 from communicable diseases.

5

Health Systems in the Service of Peace

While examining military priorities in regard to germ research, CAE has repeatedly claimed that attention should be focused on the actual crises in global public health, rather than on phantom crises promoted by the military, government, and other institutions that profit by "going along with the gag." CAE opens this chapter with a brief overview of actual world health problems. Giving exact statistics on the number of deaths from a given disease is difficult, but the reader will get the idea through the approximations below, which we think unequivocally demonstrate that nothing short of a preventable holocaust is occurring. The statistics do vary. That is in part due to the inability of poorer countries to keep accurate records, and in part due to differing systems for counting deaths (e.g., whether deaths due to tuberculosis in AIDS patients are counted as due to tuberculosis or to

AIDS or double counted). With these provisos, it can be said that globally, acute respiratory infections (including pneumonia and influenza) are the leading cause of death due to infectious agents, with over 4 million per year. Diarrheal diseases claim another 3-4 million every year. Epidemic viral diarrhea (mainly rotavirus) accounts for 873,000 per year (even though mortality in developed countries is less than one percent). Shigella causes 654,000 deaths per year; typhoid fever 581,000; intestinal amoebiasis between 40,000 and 110,000; and cholera 20,000. Most of the remainder of deaths due to diarrheal illness is due to certain strains of *E. coli* associated with contaminated water supplies in developing countries. AIDS, if one includes deaths due to tuberculosis in AIDS patients, comes next with 2.5 million. If one includes the combination TB/AIDS deaths, tuberculosis is easily the leading cause of death due to a single organism, with about 2 million every year. Malaria and measles each claim 1 million to 1.5 million per year, while hepatitis B kills between 1 million and 2 million per year. These figures are almost unintelligible because the actual quantity is so far beyond experience.

CAE is not saying that this disaster in world health is due solely to germ warfare programs hogging all the resources. Many of the problems, particularly the diarrheal illnesses, happen primarily because of capitalism's unshakable commitment to the production of poverty. People packed together in ghettos with improper water and sewage treatment is the root cause. The maddening part is that hygiene conditions are easy to change. While developed nations make some effort to alleviate this health problem, they do not do anywhere near enough. The overwhelming majority of diarrheal illness victims are the poorest, most invisible, and most powerless populations in developing countries. Knowing there will be no resistance or penalty, capitalism does its gruesome work of eliminating these surplus populations by sheer neglect. Having created engines of production that could easily end this level of poverty with a modest redistribution of wealth, the vectors of power simply ignore the issue and focus the engines of capital on producing more wealth for the wealthy and more poverty for most of the world.

To return to the diseases that are significant to this discourse (influenza, malaria, HIV, tuberculosis, and hepatitis B): not one of these top-end killers make the military's A list and, hence, are not of much interest within the scientific community funded by the military or by those researching "profitable" drugs. The problem is that medical research is a zero-sum game. Resources are finite. Only so many labs, funds, and personnel capable of doing the research exist. With so many dying every day, no nation can afford to focus its attention on nonrepresentative and improbable health issues. Nor can it focus health services solely on developing the most marketable, profitable, and/or cost effective products, leaving all else as "orphan" products. In pharmaceuticals, for example, psychiatric, erection, and heart drugs should not be the leading categories of drug development. Obviously, they are the most profitable because they are aimed at the needs and desires of the wealthy, but they do nothing to relieve the real global health crises. These are the conditions where we see the truly despotic face of capitalism. No death toll can be high enough to put people before profits.

The U.S. military and government attempt to reassure the public by claiming that benefits for all will spin off military research. We are often treated to disingenuous promissory rhetoric like the following statement on biodefense from National Institute of Allergy and Infectious Disease (NIAID) Director Anthony Fauci:

> *Furthermore, we anticipate that investments in biodefense research will have many positive spin-offs similar to the manner in which HIV/AIDS research has advanced the understanding and treatment of many other diseases. NIAID research on organisms with bioterror potential will almost certainly lead to an enhanced knowledge of other more common and naturally occurring infectious disease that afflict people around the world. In particular, the advancement of knowledge should have enormous positive effects on our ability to diagnose, treat, and prevent major diseases such as malaria, tuberculosis, HIV/AIDS, and a spectrum of emerging and reemerging diseases such as West Nile virus, dengue, and influenza.*

United States citizens have heard this doubletalk before, but in economic terms. The one lesson learned from the Reagan administration's claim of the "trickle down" effect is that making wealthy people wealthier does not help the poor. The redistribution of wealth in America has favored the wealthy for the past fifty years and only worsens with each administration. The same is true of military research on germs. As long as ebola, smallpox, anthrax, and rabbit fever are at the top of the list, little or nothing of help to the global health crisis will result. Giving the military the benefit of the doubt, suppose a useful spin-off technology was actually to occur. All well and good, but think what might have happened had that money been used for civilian-based medical initiatives to begin with? Could a cure for AIDS be better approached? Bluntly put, there is no war dividend! Civil society will not benefit from this research, and the only real hope for the poor who primarily suffer the tortures of pestilence is that they somehow fall into the category of being a U.S. "security interest."

What Is to Be Done?

The foundational answer is quite simple: The military should be banned from any participation in health issues. Health and medical research should be done in the civilian sector, and the military should get the spin-offs. Not another cent should be spent on the military's wasteful ventures. In matters of public health and public protection, the military is not needed because it does more harm than good.

Sensible plans have been around for years, but they are rejected whenever they emerge. For example, in 1990 a conference was held in Külungsborn, Germany. At this small but influential conference, Erhard Geissler suggested the idea of "Vaccines for Peace." The core of this particular idea is flawed. As we saw in chapter 4, stockpiling vaccines against the perceived threat of biological weapons is little more than a wasteful publicity stunt. Vaccines alone would offer only minimal protection from any such bug in the age of transgenics, and not everyone can be vaccinated for all known diseases on a global scale. Be that as it may, the notion of "Vaccines for Peace" has many compelling satellite ideas. First and foremost is that the military should be disinvested of any connection to vaccine research. All vaccine research should be in civilian hands. Geissler reasoned the main advantage that would emerge from this action is that the justified national and international public suspicion that the military is creating offensive capability bioweaponry would dissipate. Vaccine programs in civilian hands would be completely transparent—nothing would be classified or secret. This would in turn strengthen treaty relations and be a first step toward proper verification. (An additional advantage, which Geissler did not argue, is that it would help to keep the military out of civilian agencies such as the National Institutes of Health and the Centers for Disease Control.)

A second key idea linked to the Vaccines for Peace Program is that a vaccination program must function on a global scale. The odious link between militarism and nationalism is a hazard to public health. In the case of germ warfare, the undisputed principle of "defend America first" makes its defense almost impossible. The best way to protect the United States or any other nation against disease is to aggressively eradicate it globally through the use of all means at hand—vaccines, antibiotics, clean water programs, antipoverty initiatives, hospital and clinic proliferation, etc. The smaller the list of potential diseases for weaponization gets, the safer everyone is. Instead of wasting billions each year on useless technology and vaccines earmarked only for disposal and replacement, the United States could functionally use those billions to help those that need it most while at the same time providing for a common defense. To be sure, such an action would not completely eliminate the threat of germ warfare, but progress toward further reducing its likelihood would certainly be made, and the overall health care structure would be better prepared for any type of health crisis.

Even though many scientists rallied to the idea of civilian controlled vaccine programs, the military did not. It didn't even have to give a reason for why it objected. Biodefense, by definition, is a military operation. The military kept its germs and its vaccination programs. NATO agreed with the United States, the United Kingdom, and Germany in denouncing Vaccines for Peace, so the initiative went no further. The epilogue is sad. Rather than embracing a significant movement toward peace and health, military programs were expanded, beginning with Clinton pushing the funding for "biological defensive research" into the billions, followed by Bush refusing to sign the verification protocols in the BWC, and the ballooning expansion of the germ warfare program under his administration. Little room exists for anything other than irredeemable pessimism. In contradiction to capital's stated principles, sane, humanistic policies are rejected in favor of those of waste, uselessness, and sacrifice.

Another visionary promoting civilian control is microbiologist Mark Wheelis of the University of California, Davis. His interest is global epidemiological surveillance. He has proposed a global disease detection network constructed on four layers: a system of reporting, a system for rapid-response lab and field testing, a system for origin analysis, and an open database of medical records in order to maintain a baseline and to extrapolate patterns of disease. While he came to this notion as a means for detecting and distinguishing between natural and hostile disease outbreaks, he quickly came to see that it would better serve a generalized civilian purpose, leaving hostile detection as a small part. Even though his plan originated with military objectives in mind, Wheelis did not fall for the nationalist fallacy. He knew that disease control and biodefense have to be done on an international scale, or they are simply wasted efforts. He suggested that this global disease detection network be run by the United Nations in collaboration with the World Health Organization and the

Food and Agricultural Organization. Will a military-free network such as the one Wheelis suggests ever exist? It seems very unlikely, considering that the BWC couldn't even produce a verification protocol. That convention was the only hope to date for an international monitoring body, to be called the Organization for the Prohibition of Biological Weapons. The calls for such an organization are still being made, yet remain unanswered.

Civilian Detection in Action

While we do not have examples of the deployment of civilian agencies to cope with the fallout from a biological attack, we can examine some real scenarios that approximate a biological attack in the real world (and not as computerized or dramaturgical simulations). The most recent example is Severe Acute Respiratory Syndrome (SARS). The outbreak of SARS nearly rivals smallpox in infectiousness (SARS is not quite as contagious as smallpox). Unlike smallpox, no vaccines or known treatments were available, and the virus had not even been identified at the time of outbreak.

As a new human virus, SARS could be said to have some parallels to an attack with a transgenic bacteria or virus. Civilian agencies responded to SARS as a global civilian health crisis. The success of this response is quite remarkable. The first case of SARS was reported on November 17, 2002 in southern China. SARS became a serious problem by March 2003. On March 12 the World Health Organization issued a global alert about a "new infectious disease." On March 15 the warning was elevated after cases in Singapore and Canada were reported.

A rare emergency travel advisory was added, along with a case definition. On March 17, an international network of laboratories was formed. It had two primary missions: to identify the disease and to develop treatments. By March 24, the Centers for Disease Control presented evidence that SARS was probably a coronavirus. On April 12, Canadian researchers announced that they had sequenced the genome of the coronavirus believed to be SARS. On April 16, the new coronavirus was confirmed as the cause of SARS, according to Koch's postulates. (The germ must be present in every case of the disease; the germ must be isolated from the host with the disease and grown in pure culture; the specific disease must be reproduced when a pure culture of the germ is inoculated into a healthy susceptible host; the germ must be recoverable from the experimentally infected host.) The strategy for controlling the outbreak was to quarantine those who had the disease, or those who were believed to have been exposed to it. By July 8, the crisis was over with minimal loss of life.

No panic ensued, nor did any rushes on hospitals occur. The reason everything went smoothly was that a global generalized health plan was in place for containing infectious disease. Had militarism and nationalism accompanied it, the likelihood of serious outbreak would only have increased: information and treatments would have been classified, for example, precluding international research cooperation and a networked containment strategy. According to the military's logic, an enemy (even if inactive) can never know what is being done to fight a given disease. Research would have been limited to secure U.S. and allied labs. A probability exists that some of the most qualified researchers and medical personnel would not have been able to work on the project because of lack of the proper security status. The military is only concerned with the best strategy within a given theater of war, rather than with what will save the most people. Often, these two frames of reference are incompatible.

If anyone needs an example of what happens to public health when the military gets involved, one need look no further than the sad story of the Federal Emergency Management Agency (FEMA). Launched in 1979 by the Carter Administration, FEMA was an attempt to unify a number of federal agencies charged with managing a variety of public emergencies. These included natural disasters, nuclear war, enemy attack on U.S. territory, and incidents involving civil unrest. The Reagan Administration decided that FEMA would be most useful if it focused on civil unrest. To this end, the administration appointed former National Guard general and counter-insurgency expert Louis O. Giuffrida to the post of Emergency Czar. He, in turn, appointed more military men who shared his McCarthyist tendencies. The militarization of FEMA reached its peak in 1982 with the publication of "The Civil/Military Alliance in Emergency Management." This document contained the plans to cement the association between FEMA and the military and went on to argue for the countermanding of the constitution by saying that military force can and should be used in cases of domestic disturbances. The Reagan Administration supported this notion with several National Security Decision Directives that not only bonded FEMA to the military, but to the National Security Council as well. During this time, the Civil Security Division of FEMA pursued all kinds of nastiness including organizing military training for police and opening files on United States activists. They collected 12,000 files in all. At this point, FEMA was beginning to crowd other agencies' territories—most notably those of the FBI. In retaliation, the FBI launched a full-scale investigation of FEMA, exposing the *de facto* nepotism and misappropriation of funds. Giuffrida was forced to resign.

After this point, FEMA fell into relative neglect, and the ties to the military eroded. During this period an "all hazards disaster preparedness" plan emerged, designed so a single plan could be used to accommodate many types of emergencies. FEMA was reborn after its performance in Hurricane Andrew in 1992. The storm was the worst to have ever hit the United States and leveled parts of South Florida. This storm put a scare into both the government and the public, making it abundantly clear that the focus of FEMA should be on natural disasters that were occurring with steady or increasing (depending on who one wants to believe) regularity. In this climate, the Clinton Administration appointed James Lee Witt to be the director of the agency. For the first and only time in its history, FEMA had a director who was a professional emergency manager! Witt committed FEMA to natural disaster preparedness and disaster mitigation–quite a shift from the Reagan/Bush era.

However, this Dr. Jekyll and Mr. Hyde story does not end here. With the 2000 election of the Bush Administration, FEMA went retrograde. The Bush Administration followed through with very little of Witt's work and appointed cronies with no emergency experience (much like nominating Wolfowitz to head the World Bank even though he has no banking experience, or appointing Bolton as the ambassador to the United Nations even though he has no diplomatic experience). The Bush Administration's choice for director was Joseph Allbaugh, the former Chief of Staff for Governer Bush and the former national campaign manager for the Bush-Cheney campaign.

Allbaugh resigned in 2003. His buddy and GOP activist Mike Brown, who had been appointed Deputy Director when Allbaugh joined FEMA in 2001, succeeded him. Like Allbaugh, Brown had no experience in emergency management.

After 9/11, the administration decided that FEMA was an anachronism, the duties of which should fall under the new Department of Homeland Security. Public protection from natural disasters once again shifted back toward the military, and the only disaster that garnered government attention in the post 9/11 climate was terrorism. Once again, military paranoia rather than public health became the order of the day. Under Brown, FEMA developed a new "all hazards" plan suitable only for the many types of terrorist attacks that the agency could dream up. Public health emergency equipment was replaced with military first response equipment for WMDs. Given the catastrophe in New Orleans and the Gulf Coast in 2005, the consequences of this shift are clear. An underfunded and unprepared FEMA attempted to manage the greatest natural disaster in United States history. (The scope of the disaster was massive in part due to the diverting of preparedness funds to the war in Iraq, particularly those for infrastructure such as levees). The military was almost completely useless, giving little support until nearly a week after the storm hit. The many casualties were not from the storm, but from the sheer incompetence of the Bush Administration to ensure funding for the necessary precautions against such a disaster, in combination with the inhuman negligence of authorities and the unpreparedness of FEMA. The clear lesson here, once again, is that a militarized relationship to public health serves only to intensify disaster and not to lessen it.

Another scenario about which the Bush Administration and the military often fantasize is the poisoning of the food supply. A terrorist could set loose a fungus that would kill our crops, or a food could be directly infected with *E. coli*, salmonella, or worse. Both of these possibilities are actually common natural threats to public health. Disease management in crops is fairly standard, as it is in animals, and is done quite successfully. Food processing is also a managed situation with many interlocking layers of inspection, and for the most part, such precautions have worked very well in ensuring public safety. The United States has had two public health problems from food in recent years, both stemming from the distribution of tainted hamburger. The first was at a Jack in the Box restaurant in Washington State in 1993 in which approximately 100 people became ill, resulting in one death. The second had to do with a meatpacking incident at the ConAgra distribution plant in Colorado in 2002. *E. coli 0157:H7* got into the meat as in the Jack in the Box incident, but since this occurred at a major distributor's packing plant it lead to the recall of nearly 19 million pounds of ground beef. Of this 19 million pounds, most was consumed rather than returned.

This would seem like a perfect terrorist plot. A single person could get a job at a meat packing plant and poison the meat with naturally occurring bacteria. The meat would then be distributed throughout the United States. No one would even suspect it was terrorism until responsibility was claimed. For that matter, a terrorist cell or network could claim responsibility even if it was a natural occurrence. Although natural in origin, what happened with ConAgra parallels such a situation, and the body count was only one, along with a few dozen illnesses.

The food industry has consistently fought an annual legal battle against any USDA safety control, preferring instead to police itself. The Bush administration has agreed with this policy and rolled back what legislation it could, in addition to stacking the USDA with officers sympathetic to meat and livestock interests. The USDA Secretary for Congressional Relations was a former ConAgra employee, and the chief of staff for the Secretary of Agriculture, Dale Moore, was a former lobbyist for the National Cattleman's Beef Association. Even with these problems, Americans do not seem to be afraid of eating a rare hamburger and should not be. Federal standards are not the only ones in place. State standards also offer protection, in addition to our own ability to spot tainted meat or to thoroughly cook it as many restaurants do. Obviously, food corporations do not want to poison their customers. That is not good for business. They want to be protected against liability if an accident happens. In spite of all its imperfections, the health system as a whole seems to work in regard to food and its distribution.

The point is that whether it is disease or other matters of the organic realm, the civilian sector is better capable of protecting public health than is the military. The politics are simple: the civilian sector has civilian interests at heart; the military has military interests at heart. The interests are not the same.

Natural Pressures

The highest probability of a disaster due to disease is from influenza—not so much the strains of flu that regularly occur during the winter months, but a new form to which humans have little or no immunity. The last time such a flu emerged was in autumn 1918. The hygienic conditions were perfect, given the cramped and soiled conditions in which soldiers were living at the end of World War I. Add this hygienic problem to a similar one among pigs that were in contact with some of the soldiers (primarily kitchen staff), and the stage was set. In 1918, the flu jumped from pigs to humans. What further fanned the flames of this disaster was the fact that troops and pigs were being moved around on an international scale, so not only was the problem one of environment, but the perfect conditions for vector movement also existed, allowing for maximum efficiency in the distribution of the virus (given the relative scale of mass human movement at that time in history). The result was approximately 25 million deaths worldwide, with close to one million deaths in the United States.

Influenza viruses can mutate at an incredible rate and, on rare occasion, can develop the ability to jump species. The usual path to people is from birds to pigs to humans. If conditions are good, not only can the virus develop the capacity to jump to humans, but it may also develop the capacity to spread from human to human once it completes its species advance. At this point, the disaster begins. Since the virus is one that evolved in birds, human bodies have not interacted with the virus before and hence have no natural immuno-defenses against it. Currently, the primary candidate to repeat the 1918 health crisis is avian flu. This flu has jumped from bird to human, cutting out the middleman (pigs), and has resulted in nearly 100 deaths. Those likely to acquire this disease are people working with poultry in less-than-sanitary conditions. Whether it will ever spread from human to human is unknown, but the potential is there.

The good news is that unlike a terror attack, authorities can see this problem coming and can begin to specifically prepare for it or at least to include it in an "all hazards disaster preparedness" plan. The bad news is that preparedness of this sort is not likely to happen. One reason is that the military has little interest in this germ, and another is that, as discussed earlier, the Bush administration has little interest in maintaining even the inadequate public healthcare system now in place. On every medical front, the United States and the world are facing increasingly deteriorating health conditions due to the current administration's recklessness. With regard to catastrophe coming from disease, the United States is failing in every department—research, preparedness, organization, finances, and almost anything else that can be imagined. In every case, the wrong choices are being made at taxpayer expense, and it is because of the military's overwhelming influence on the decisions being made by the government, as well as the Bush Administration's propensity for military solutions to crisis situations.

A General Strike

If only the ideal were possible. A general strike of all scientists in the life sciences, unified by the demand that disease research and preparedness should be solely civilian-based, would eventually bring the United States and the world to a far less precarious place. A singular scientific technocracy has that kind of power, because its members are necessary and irreplaceable. Unfortunately, money can make the pain of a guilty conscience quite tolerable, leaving the above vision as useless as weaponized germs. A possible resistance in this arena of politics does not have to take an extreme form, but it does have to be ongoing and popular. For this to happen, the general public must be made aware that even "defensive" germ warfare programs expose individuals to unacceptable dangers instead of making them more secure, and these programs are an obscene waste of tax dollars and public resources. The choice of military interests over public health interests is a sure recipe for disaster, and this is not a fantasy like the terrorist scenario. This view is an undeniable fact demonstrated by the millions who are dying every year and by the historical record on epidemics and military exploits in the public sphere.

Uncontrolled emerging infectious disease is an ongoing nightmare that will only intensify in the future. If a popular front can be constructed around the demand to keep the military out of public health policy, institutions, and initiatives, then activists, cultural producers, and concerned citizens can begin to do the impossible: discourage scientists from working for or with the military; force pharmaceutical companies to make antibiotics and vaccines that combat the diseases that are killing people; remove all germ research from the military and redirect the funds to civilian initiatives; force the signing of verification protocols; and have all disease research declassified so that it can be used in the public interest on a global scale. Once again, people must join together to invert the most vicious and horrific first principle of capital—profits before people must become people before profits.

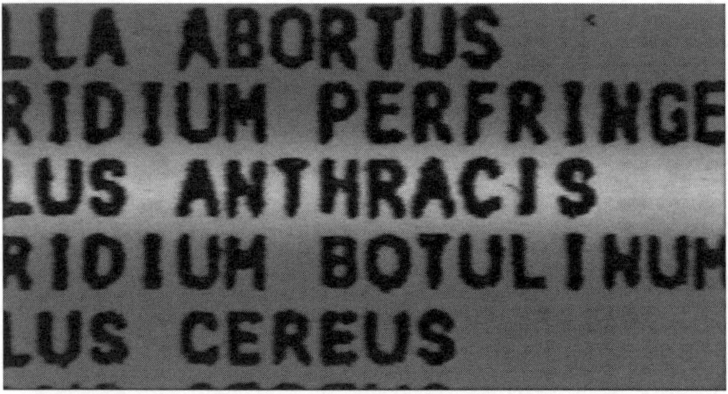

Inventory detail of sale to Saddam Hussein. From 1985 until 1990 the U.S. government approved 771 licenses [only 39 were rejected] for the export to Iraq of $1.5 billion worth of biological agents and high-tech equipment with military applications. The American Type Culture Collection made 70 shipments of the anthrax bug and other pathogenic agents.

Appendix I

When Thought Becomes Crime[1]

Critical Art Ensemble

How Did it Come to This?

Only a perverse authoritarian logic can explain how CAE can at one moment be creating the project "Free Range Grain" for the *At Your Own Risk* exhibition at Schirn Kunsthalle in Frankfurt, reconfiguring it for *The Interventionists* exhibition at Mass MoCA in a second moment, and then suddenly have a CAE member in FBI detention. The U.S. Justice Department has accused us of such shocking crimes as bioterrorism, health and safety violations, mail fraud, wire fraud, and even murder. Now, as we retool "Free Range Grain" for the *Risk* exhibition at the Glasgow Center for Contemporary Art, the surreal farce of our legal nightmare continues unabated.

Of course, we always knew that cultural interventionist work could have serious consequences. And over the years, predictably, CAE has been denounced (and threatened) by all varieties of authority: cops, corporate lawyers, politicians, all types of racists, and church groups—even the Archbishop of Salzburg. But to be the target of an international investigation that involves the FBI; the Joint Terrorism Task Force; the ATF; the Department of Homeland Security; the Department of Health and Safety; numerous local police agencies; and even Canadian, Norwegian, and German federal investigators goes far beyond the pale. As of this writing, CAE member Steven Kurtz, and one of our long-time collaborators, University of Pittsburgh geneticist Robert Ferrell, are fighting the insanely real threat of being sent to federal prison.

So how did we create such a vortex of Kafkaesque legalistic repression? In the "Free Range Grain" project, for instance, CAE simply used molecular biology techniques to test for genetically modified food in the global food trade. We want(ed) this interventionist performance to demonstrate how the "smooth space" of global trade enables the very "contaminations" the authorities say it guards against. Now we, along with our colleagues on the CAE defense team, have been trying to understand why the authorities have taken such a reactionary position in regard to our art practice. We have come up with many reasons; we can address only a few in this brief article.

The first reason, we believe, involves the discourse in which we framed our project. By viewing the scientific process through the lens of the capitalist political economy, we disrupted the legitimized version of science as a self-contained, value-free specialization. The powers that be would have science speak for itself, within and about itself. This insularity is akin to Clement Greenberg's idea of letting art history explain the production of art, or Emile Durkheim's use of "social facts" to explain the social. But any discourse exists within larger historical and political contexts. It seemed self-evident for us to place competing discourses in conversation, and to show the socioeconomic ideologies at work in food production. From the perspective of authority, however, we were being subversive, deviant. For those who wish to preserve the autonomy of science, citizens can discuss scientific structure, method, materials, etc., as long as they do not refer to the political or economic interests that impinge on scientific research. A biology club can talk about cells, but if it goes beyond the institutionalized boundaries of the life sciences, look out for the feds.

The second challenge we posed came from our amateur approach to life-science knowledge systems, experimental processes, acquisition of materials, etc. An amateur can be critical of an institution without fear of recrimination or loss of status or investment. An art professor, for example, will probably not tell students that art school is a pyramid scheme into which they will pour a lot of capital, feed the higher-ups, and probably get very little if anything in return. That criticism is more likely to emerge from outside the power structure (or from disgruntled ex-students). In science, where the financial stakes are much higher, any criticism of resources may well result in funding cuts—a situation one can ill afford in such a capital-intensive discipline. So it takes an outsider to science—a creative tinkerer—to rattle the cage of the discipline's most dearly held assumptions and practices.

With special regard to the institutional financing of science, the amateur reveals the profit-driven privatization of a discipline that is purportedly—mythologically—open to all. By undertaking research as if science were truly a forum in which all may participate according to their abilities and resources, CAE angers those who manipulate scientific activity through capital investment. The financial stakes are so high that the authorities can imagine only one motivation for critical, amateur research, particularly if it is conducted at home outside of systems of surveillance/discipline. If that research intends to expose, disrupt, or subvert the meta-narratives that put scientific investigation in the service of profit, the amateur investigator must want to produce terrorist acts.

In the paranoid political climate of the United States, American authorities leap all too easily from ideological criticism to terrorism. Moreover, CAE's legal battle reveals that the government has made thinking into a crime: a citizen can be arrested without having committed any act of terror or without having done anything illegal at all. Former U.S. Attorney General John Ashcroft has unofficially reformed law enforcement policy and practice according to the Bush administration's idea of "preemptive war." He has argued that if indicators—any type of dissent in relation to the interests of the investing classes or "national interest"—suggest that a person or group could do something illegal, then they should be arrested, detained, deported, or otherwise persecuted with the full resources of all repressive state agencies. Apparently, the U.S. Justice Department is now trying to make CAE into an example of what can happen to citizens whose only "crime" is having thoughts of dissent enacted within the sphere of legality and with the alleged protection of constitutional rights.

For experimental art, political art, tactical media, and independent media in the United States (and to some degree in other nations), the implications of Steven Kurtz's arrest are profound. The repressive forces of the state are directly targeting producers of cultural interventionist work. In past decades, policymakers have often leaned on political artwork through financial penalties such as rescinding artist's grants, folding federal arts programs, and economically squeezing out the spaces that exhibit subversive work.[2] Now, these attacks on civil grounds have undergone a horrific paradigm shift, and individual artists are being charged with criminal activity. The persecution works slowly and insidiously, through silencing artists, looting their work and their research, and constraining their movement. We are no longer seeing cultural conflict in action, but a proto-fascist attack upon open source management of expression itself.

---

[1] The set of theses presented in this document were collectively developed through a series of lectures given by the CAE defense team. Contributors include Doug Ashford, Gregg Bordowitz, CAE, Natalie Jeremijenko, Claire Pentecost, and Lucia Sommer. Special thanks to Karen Schiff for editing.

[2] The New York Council for the Humanities recently rescinded a grant awarded to the City University of New York for its series on academic freedom because Steve Kurtz was one of the invited speakers!

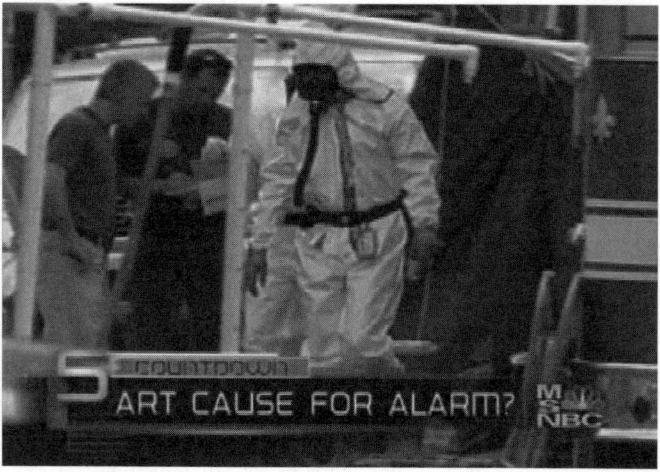

Art cause for alarm!

Appendix II

Reflections on the Case by the U.S. Justice Department against Steven Kurtz and Robert Ferrell

Claire Pentecost[1]

Many people have asked us why the Justice Department is pursuing this case.

Meaning, when the Buffalo Health Department affirmed there was nothing dangerous in the Kurtz home and that Hope Kurtz died of natural causes, when the FBI saw that the possession of scientific equipment and materials in Kurtz's home studio was completely consistent with his practice as an artist and that his practice has a long, public, and institutionally validated record, then, why didn't they drop the case? When it became clear even through the Grand Jury investigation that this was not a case of bioterrorism, why did they pursue it? Couldn't they see that Critical Art Ensemble's work is art?

As often as not the questioners answer their own question, saying it must be a matter of saving face: the Justice Department (DOJ) now has to justify the time and money they spent on this case in the first few weeks and has to answer to the publicity the case has attracted.

An overview of prosecutions since 9/11 originating with suspicion of terrorism suggests the department has a different logic for evaluating its results than might first be apparent to the public. And "saving face" is not at the top of the list.

Bad Company

One can imagine that investigative agencies and U.S. attorneys are under enormous pressure to produce results in the "War on Terror." To put it crudely, in the last three-and-a-half years, probably nothing has influenced promotions and funding more. Less crudely, there are no doubt many dedicated people in the Justice Department genuinely concerned to prevent more terrorist events large or small. But like most of the Bush administration, this department manages to account for itself by its own warped calculations, while a typically meretricious press and a complicit public have all but spared U.S. Justice the shame of its waste, incompetence, and brutal racism.

Numbers of such cases and their outcome are difficult to put together accurately for several reasons, most prominently that the Justice Department has ceased publishing its data. Also, after 9/11, for its internal record keeping, the department created many new categories of crimes it considered terrorist, most significantly an umbrella category called, confusingly enough, "Anti-Terrorism," which is "intended to prevent or disrupt potential or actual terrorist threats where the offense conduct is not obviously a federal crime of terrorism."[2] This category includes immigration, identity theft, drug, and like cases. In short, the domestic version of preemptive strike. And then there is the problem that the DOJ may be distorting the figures it does release: in January 2003 the General Accounting Office reported that at least 46 percent of all terrorism-related convictions for FY 2002 were misclassified, and of cases alleged to meet the qualifications for international terrorism, a minimum of 75 percent did not. As a consequence one finds a variety of numbers published, for instance:

David Cole, legal affairs correspondent for *The Nation*[3] tells us that since 9/11, of over 5,000 foreign nationals detained by Ashcroft's department on suspicion of terrorism, exactly none have been convicted of terrorism. Many detainees have been indicted for routine violations involving immigration, fraud, laundering, and identity theft. On the one hand it would seem that the Justice Department has devised some new tools to help the INS sweep for visa problems. On the other hand, it seems the INS and the Social Security Administration are becoming as important as the FBI in referring cases of possible terrorism to the DOJ.[4]

Transactional Records Access Clearinghouse (TRAC), an independent analyzer of federal records based at Syracuse University, reports that in the two years following 9/11, Federal investigators (primarily the FBI) recommended 6,400 matters for prosecution by the government either related to suspicion of having committed terrorist acts or on charges that fit the new "Anti-Terrorism" category described above. By September

30, 2003, the government had processed 2,681 of these cases. A total of five had been sentenced to twenty years or more in prison. In the category of international terrorists, the median sentence was 14 days.[5] These kinds of punishments do not suggest that for all the people being investigated and dragged through the system, serious terrorists are being snagged.

At the March 2003 hearings before the Senate Judiciary Committee, Ashcroft boasted that his 9/11 investigations had led to 478 deportations. It was not mentioned that most of these were for visa violations, and that in fact the FBI must clear deportees of suspicion of terrorism *before* deporting them. Maybe some of these were illegal deportations to the offshore torture centers we have learned about since cases like that of Maher Arar have begun to surface. Arar, a Syrian-born Canadian citizen, was detained by U.S. agents at Kennedy Airport in September 2002. Without being charged, he was sent to Syria where he spent a year in prison being tortured and interrogated. He was released in October 2003 after Canadian authorities intervened on his behalf. He is now suing the U.S. government.[6]

What is going on here? Let's look at the kinds of cases we do know about.

If we were to group them loosely, we could make one class of cases that actually do bring quite a bit of evidence to accuse alleged terrorists of attempted acts or plots. An example might be Richard Reid, the "shoe bomber," who was caught in the act, pleaded guilty to attempting to blow up a plane, swore allegiance to bin Laden and denounced U.S. policy at his sentencing hearing, where he received a life sentence. Another might be Zacarias Moussaoui, the so-called "twentieth hijacker" because he swears allegiance to al Qaeda, went to flight school in the United States and at one time received money from operatives who financed some of the other hijackers. His trial has been stalled for two years as he fights to call key witnesses whom he claims could testify that he knew nothing of the plot. The potential witnesses, Ramzi Binalshibh, Mustafa Ahmed al-Hawsawi, and Khalid Shaikh Mohammed, designated "enemy combatants," are in custody in undisclosed locations in other countries, and the U.S. government maintains that their participation in Moussaoui's trial even via videotape would "cause irreparable harm to the war on al Qaeda." Because the same witnesses were also denied by the United States in the defense of Mounir el Mottasadeq, the only defendant tried as part of the Hamburg cell of the 9/11 hijackers, a German judge has declared his conviction invalid and called for a new trial.

The second group, by far the largest, is the notoriously abused company, mostly men of Arabic origin and/or Islamic faith, arrested or detained with what appears to be a complete lack of evidence or regard for civil rights, and ultimately a complete lack of a case related to terrorism. Most of these remain nameless to the general public but some became high profile bungles of U.S. Justice. Here we can include Brandon Mayfield, the Muslim Attorney wrongly accused of the Madrid subway bombing because of a grossly mismatched fingerprint, secretly investigated under provisions of the PATRIOT Act and jailed for two weeks. Or Jose Padilla, a Chicago ex-convict, convert to Islam, and al Qaeda wannabe,[7] held for almost three years without charges in a Naval brig. In February 2005, a judge in the 2nd Circuit ruled the President did not have the power to hold a U.S. citizen as an "enemy combatant" and ordered Padilla released, but on September 9, 2005, a federal appeals court upheld the power of the president to indefinitely detain so-called enemy combatants, including U.S. citizens, without any charges.

Certainly there are more and longer stories to tell about the abuses against specific Muslim men, but for the purposes of this paper, it's the numbers and the general disregard for evidence of terrorist connections that make this category significant. This is where we find the domestic sweeps: over 5,000 effectively random detainees, the prosecutions and deportations of men who have worked and raised families in this country for years. Then the international sweeps: the 600 uncharged and unrepresented men subjected to torture in Guantanamo after being picked up in Afghanistan or elsewhere.

In order to understand more about what is happening in the Kurtz-Ferrell case, we can identify a third class of cases, in which the rhetoric of terrorism and the expanded juridical toolbox for fighting it are being used to punish and intimidate critics of U.S. policy whether they are Islam-identified or not. In some cases, this is accomplished by turning small infractions into crimes precisely because the defendant can be associated with beliefs very unpopular in a time of national hysteria. In other cases, it's done by exposing a suspect to humiliating investigation and expensive legal defense over charges that finally come to nothing.

Here we might list Captain James Yee, the Muslim army chaplain charged with serving the detainees at Guantanamo Bay. When he advocated against their illegal and inhumane treatment, he was accused of espionage, but the outcome of a lengthy investigation and a legal battle that cost the defendant over

$160,000 was that the Army reprimanded him for downloading internet porn and committing adultery. Or we might look at the case of University of South Florida Computer Science professor Sami al-Arian. Because he ran an Islamic think-tank and a Palestinian advocacy group in the 1990s, the FBI pursued a 10-year investigation trying to assemble evidence that he provided material support to terrorist organizations. Even though the FBI raided his office and home, his university conducted a separate investigation, and a judge re-examined the charges in 2000, no incriminating evidence was found. In the post-9/11 frenzy to prove their diligence, the U.S. Justice Department renewed their investigation and indicted al-Arian for conspiracy in February 2003.[8]

Sherman Austin, leftist activist and founder of www.raisethefist.org (a website hosting a number of leftist groups' webpages), was investigated for having a link on his site to Reclaim Guide, which offers information on explosives. Though the information was minimal compared with what can be found in countless libraries and websites, notably white supremacist websites, Austin was sentenced for "distribution" of information about making or using explosives with the "intent" that such information "be used for, or in furtherance of, an activity that constitutes a Federal crime of violence." He served a year in federal prison. Under U.S. First Amendment protection, publishing, distributing, reading, thinking about, or talking about such information cannot constitute a crime. Under the current U.S. justice system, it can be construed as criminal if it is associated with beliefs critical of the government, in which case the perpetrator deserves a pre-emptive strike.

Manlin Chee, a naturalized American citizen and an immigration lawyer who represented many poor and Muslim immigrants, was awarded the 1991 American Bar Association service award, presented to her by Justice Sandra Day O'Connor. When she became an outspoken critic of the USA PATRIOT Act, the FBI began an investigation of her practice. After a year of pouring through documents on three decades of her cases, interviewing her clients and employees, and constructing a sting operation with agents posing as needy Muslims trying to obtain papers on questionable grounds, the FBI had her indicted for immigration fraud. Under pressure, Chee pled guilty and on March 3, 2005 she was sentenced to a year in jail.

It's hard to know just how much the USA PATRIOT Act is being used in investigations because part of the power of "sneak and peek" is that the law never has to disclose the wiretaps, searches, surveillances, or DNA swabs they may have deemed necessary to determine suspicion.[9] But, at the level of the courts, we are seeing an earlier, less-publicized law become a handy prosecutor's hammer. Among other provisions, "The Antiterrorism and Effective Death Penalty Act of 1996," signed by Clinton after the Oklahoma City bombing, renders it a crime for U.S. citizens to provide material support to the lawful political or humanitarian activities of any foreign group designated by the Secretary of State as "terrorist."

A tragic case delivering convictions in 2003 on the basis of the material support argument is that of six young Yemeni Americans from the defunct steel town of Lackawanna, New York. Low-income, working, first- and second-generation Americans, they were recruited by a religious fundamentalist to an al Qaeda training camp in Afghanistan in the spring of 2001 where some of them actually met Osama bin Laden. Confronted with the reality of a jihadi organization, they returned home, ceasing ties with the man who recruited them (who was later killed by a U.S. Predator drone in Yemen). By all accounts they got on with their lives and never knew about, planned, or in any other way supported terrorists or terrorist actions. The travesty in this case was the severity of the punishment and the way it was won. The axe over the defense was the constant threat of being declared enemy combatants, which would deliver them to a military prison without access to lawyers, courts, or their families—possibly a life sentence by executive fiat. The prosecutors never offered evidence that the Lackawanna defendants intended to commit any act of terrorism, but under the pressure of losing all legal rights, they pled guilty and received sentences ranging from 6-1/2 to 10 years. A condition of the plea was a waiver by each defendant of the right to appeal, even if the Supreme Court were later to find the law unconstitutional.

As the 9/11 report attests, in spring 2001 Ashcroft had taken terrorism off the list of funding priorities and Condoleezza Rice didn't have the time of day for the State Department terrorism experts. Although people at the top level of government have not been held to account for being unable or unwilling to heed mounting evidence that al Qaeda would become the number one U.S. threat, six young men from Lackawanna should have known that they risked 25-year prison sentences by exploring the promises of radical forms of their religion.

With particular regard to the domestic sweeps and persecutions, even some pundits sympathetic to the "War on Terror" have pointed out that the government is violently alienating the community of U.S. Muslims whose cooperation might be useful to them. Clearly, cooperation is not a priority. "Catching terrorists" may be the advertised objective, but what these policies demonstrate is that there is a broader goal, a more urgent necessity for a larger vision. What the terrorist attacks of 9/11 represented to their target, multinational capital, embodied in the World Trade Center, and its ally, the U.S. military, embodied in the Pentagon, is that the pan-Islamic independence movement is out of control and must be eliminated. For global capital to continue to integrate one "nonintegrated" region after another, especially those with valuable resources, the notion of Islamic independence, like any vigorous third world independence movement, is in the way and must be crushed. And this means that any potential sympathizers with such a movement must be set straight. In this case, people of Islamic identification everywhere must be disciplined, must be shown that the privileges of the first world, including democracy and basic human rights, are only theirs by the discretion of first world superpowers, the United States and the European Union.

Of the Lackawanna Six, Bush boasted that the government had broken up a terrorist sleeper cell. In 2003 John Ashcroft gave the Justice Department's highest award, "The Attorney General's Award for Exceptional Service" to the members of the Buffalo Joint Terrorism Task Force for the dismantlement of the Lackawanna terrorist cell. Many of the award recipients were part of the team that conducted the investigation of Kurtz. The award-winning prosecutor who presented the case against the Yemeni Americans, William J. Hochul, Jr., is now prosecuting Steve Kurtz and Robert Ferrell. Besides heading the anti-terrorism unit in the Western District of New York State, his specialty is the use of fraud and racketeering charges in criminal cases against white collar, violent, and organized crime.

Referring to the Lackawanna case, Deputy Attorney General Larry D. Thompson said, "Terrorism and support of terrorists is not confined to large cities. It lurks in small towns and rural areas." An advantage of the Kurtz-Ferrell case is that it illustrates that U.S. Justice does not only prosecute the dark and the poor, but that it will also hunt the white and the professionally salaried. The enemy is not confined to those we easily recognize as other, but comes disguised as college professors in the arts and sciences. Justice is fair; the enemy is everywhere.

In this way, even as the architects of a privileged society wage war on a population they have deemed a threat or obstacle, they consolidate the loyalty of the included. This requires disciplining any serious criticism of the system being defended. Even in the best of times, the law is multifarious and discretionary, meaning that laws are generally enforced in an unequal manner, so that the more enfranchised, "valued" citizenry are less likely to encounter the law for the same actions that will trip the less enfranchised, generally suspected, disposable people. And this is always put to political ends, sometimes urgently when a "present danger" can be broadcast and other times more routinely. When the reigning defense moves from routine mechanisms of ideology and enforcement to broader operations of brutality, the tactics must be justified by vilifying more than just the outsiders, in fact by showing any class of detractor to be deviant and punishable.

It's easy to believe this ambitious prosecutor and his team find the content of Critical Art Ensemble's work, especially their writings, so radically deviant from their own plan for America that they consider it criminal. Everything about the art group's activity has always been completely legal, and their ideas are protected by the First Amendment. As little respect as the Bush administration shows for the U.S. Constitution or any other inconvenient law, national or international, they have not yet been able to openly trump the First Amendment.[10] But the judicial trance induced by the mantra of terrorism currently gives the prosecution supraconstitutional powers, specifically end-runs around First Amendment rights. Unfortunately, the Kurtz-Ferrell case may follow the formula of neutral infraction + leftist politics = inflation to terrorist proportions.

The Ownership Society

After the possible charge of bioterrorism against Kurtz, the charges of mail and wire fraud appeared to many as small and technical, but these are serious felonies. Two counts each of mail and wire fraud carry the same potential sentence as the original bioterrorism charge would have: up to 20 years. Charges of mail fraud and more recently wire fraud are designed to dismantle phony financial schemes that defraud the public out of money through mail, credit card, or internet. Because these laws are written very broadly, they are also used to nail figures in organized crime and, in the same way, have been used to put away social and political troublemakers such as Marcus Garvey.[11]

Exactly what transaction between Kurtz and Ferrell is alleged to be fraudulent? According to the indictment, Ferrell used his University of Pittsburgh agreement with American Type Culture Collection (ATCC) to obtain $256 worth of harmless bacteria that he then sent through the mail to Kurtz. A federal offense? Here are the details of the context:

Research and educational labs obtain biological samples from companies like ATCC through formalized agreements called Material Transfer Agreements (MTAs). Some samples are regulated because they are lethal pathogens and their handling should by all accounts be tightly controlled, but all samples are regulated as intellectual property. ATCC handles the deadliest to the most benign bacteria used in high school biology labs. To purchase any of these, one has to be part of a research or educational institution and sign a contract forbidding the buyer to sell, share, mail, or reproduce the sample. In its generic form, this is basically an intellectual property agreement designed to control a product which, once in the hands of the consumer, is infinitely reproducible. Think of the licensing agreement you accept when you open new software or the copyright agreement you enter when you buy recorded music. Apparently, in the collaborative culture of biology labs, MTAs are about as routine. They are signed by the principal investigator of a lab at a university, while researchers and bench scientists in those labs do in fact share, save, reproduce, transport, and send samples through the mail all the time. Ask a biologist.

If the defendants did what is alleged in the indictment, they broke a contract. At most, this is a civil offense to be settled between the University of Pittsburgh and ATCC, but neither of these parties have brought any complaint against Ferrell or Kurtz. To our knowledge this is the first time the U.S. Justice Department is intervening in the alleged breach of an MTA of nonhazardous materials in order to redefine it as a criminal offense.

The U.S. Department of Justice publishes a *Criminal Resource Handbook* available online, in which it states a general "Prosecution Policy Relating to Mail Fraud and Wire Fraud" as follows:

> *Prosecutions of fraud ordinarily should not be undertaken if the scheme employed consists of some isolated transactions between individuals, involving minor loss to the victims, in which case the parties should be left to settle their differences by civil or criminal litigation in the state courts. Serious consideration, however, should be given to the prosecution of any scheme which in its nature is directed to defrauding a class of persons, or the general public, with a substantial pattern of conduct.*[12]

Is the Western New York Office of the U.S. DOJ pursuing yet another Bush line of legal activism, this one a strategy to criminalize the breach of MTAs? This is a very interesting question and unanswerable. I will speculate about it anyway, but first stress again that it's more likely that Hochul & Co. primarily want to publicly punish Kurtz and Ferrell for the ideas they represent, and to sustain the campaign of intimidation against dissent. But beyond this there are aspects of the case offering other gains consistent with neoliberal and neocon priorities.

For all the myths of creative genius, different drummers, posters of Einstein's wild halo of hair backlit under an injunction to "think different," careers in science are not made by stepping out of line. More than ever the line in question is the bottom line. Research universities are increasingly expected to perform as drivers of the economy by making discoveries that are patentable and marketable in short order. Written to move new technology into the marketplace faster, the 1980 Bayh Dole Act made it easier for individual scientists and their institutions, whether public or private, to profit by patenting their own research. Add to this the 1980 Chakraborty decision legalizing the patenting of life forms, the boom in the pharmaceutical market, and twenty-five years later research universities have become the hubs of countless networks in which scientists, venture capitalists, and small companies float new technologies on the market. Many of the start-ups fail, but the successful ones are bought out by bigger companies, the whole system serving as a cost-free, R&D-to-market proving ground.

Increasingly, the universities themselves are growing dependent on the money made in their technology transfer offices where patents are handled. And corporate funding in the form of grants or partnerships is becoming a routine way to make up for shortfalls as state and federal funding shrink. This conforms neatly with the right-wing-since-Reagan agenda to privatize all activities once pursued as public stakes in a common welfare.

Privatization is clearly the shibboleth of the reigning Republican ideologues, but it's more than privatizing the military and hiring mercenaries to make possible an unpopular war, or borrowing trillions to privatize a perfectly healthy social security system. The privatization of information is now at the heart of capitalism.

In some industries this has made the difference between routine and enormous profits. In particular, the life sciences have achieved an importance well beyond the U.S. research institution. Pharmaceutical blockbusters that treat the "crotch to cranium" ills and complaints of the first world as well as the gene rush in both plant and animal forms have made the life sciences the meeting ground of multinational profiteers, global treaty disputes, and rioting farmers in the global south. Proprietary advances under what we used to call biology have become an investment frontier second only to petroleum in the waging of national security. This is an integral part of U.S. foreign policy, exercised through multi- and bilateral trade agreements insisting on conformity to intellectual property regimes granting commercial control over biodiversity, as well as over agricultural methods and resources.

What does this have to do with Critical Art Ensemble and the case against Kurtz and Ferrell?

In the direct sense, the work that has clearly made the artist so reprehensible to the U.S. Attorney's office has been dedicated to critiquing this situation for several years. In addition, the alleged breach of contract that is here being transfigured into a criminal offense is only one of the rapidly proliferating legal instruments that regulate property in our lives, especially intellectual property. An MTA may seem remote and technical, a tic in the bureaucracy of science, but it represents a growing category of actions that make the individual increasingly vulnerable to authoritarian interference in the name of property.

The more our resources, needs, pleasures, and experiences are socially and legally defined as "property," the more the state is authorized to infiltrate our lives and regulate disputes of ownership. This is happening in the realms of leisure, work and, as stated earlier, international relations. Current consumer technologies of music and image make reproduction inevitable so, as we see when high school kids are busted to make an example, legal and repressive measures are the only way to enforce ownership. In the case of transgenic seeds, farmers sign contracts foregoing the right to reproduce, save, sell, share or give away any of a product which, if used as directed, will reproduce itself. The leading holder of patents in agriculture, Monsanto, has investigated and harassed over 500 farmers in the United States for breach of this property agreement which is very similar to an MTA but with much more draconian consequences.[13] A fundamental tenet of membership in the WTO and of all U.S. and E.U. trade agreements with developing nations insists that the trading partner establish and enforce intellectual property regimes consistent with those in the global north. One of the reasons that the United States is so eager to help multinationals get transgenic agriculture rooted in the extensively rural global south is that it is practically a one-step process to drive patents and intellectual property regimes into the most basic register of their lives and economy.

The ethos of CAE's work, its process, content, and rhetoric runs counter to the elitist protection of knowledge, whether as property or as privilege. CAE assumes the role of the amateur, the energetic, engaged nonprofessional approaching a specialization such as genetics or biotechnology to expose its uses to public scrutiny. The preferred way to do this is collaboration with someone from within the field, although this is not always possible. What is happening in the legal elaboration of intellectual property is that we are either able to find a collaborator or we are forced to become thieves. In this case the implication is that even with a reputable and willing collaborator, we will be named as thieves.

At this moment, the charges are no longer related to bioterrorism, but as far as the prosecution goes, the trial will probably not be much about MTAs or the culture of biology research or the legitimacy of the amateur. The prosecutor will do his best to make it about the perversity of the saboteur. The courtroom is not so much about the law as it is about persuading the jury by any means necessary. No doubt Kurtz will be dramatized as reckless and anti-American: a combination tantamount to terrorist. Since Ferrell is a venerable scientist in his sixties currently undergoing treatment for cancer, hopefully he will not be so direct a personal target, although scientists have at least as much at stake as artists in this case.

Capital Defense

Scientists have had their own problems with the Bush administration. Some of this is evidenced in a report by the Union of Concerned Scientists called "Scientific Integrity in Policy Making" signed by over 6,000 scientists, including 48 Nobel Laureates, 62 National Medal of Science Recipients, and 127 Members of the National Academy of Sciences. It lists the many overrides of independent scientific advisories by ideology in the last four years.[14]

Another document more relevant to this case is the letter from 758 scientists to the director of the National Institutes of Health protesting the shift of tens of million of dollars in federal research money from major public health diseases to obscure pathogens the government has designated as bioterrorist threats. The scientists say that, since 2001, grants for research on the bacteria that cause anthrax and five other diseases rare or nonexistent in the United States have increased fifteenfold, while grants to study bacteria not associated with bioterrorism have decreased 27 percent. The underfunded class includes common serious germs such as tuberculosis and syphilis. The February 28, 2005 letter is posted on the website of the magazine *Science*.

This is especially germane to the case because CAE was developing projects critical of U.S. biodefense policy when the FBI raided Steve Kurtz's home. The harmless bacteria allegedly obtained under Ferrell's MTA was for a project criticizing the history of U.S. bioweapons development and testing. Many of the books the FBI confiscated were on the history of bioweapons. On Kurtz's computer, also confiscated, was part of a manuscript on the subject. What was CAE's critique almost a year ago? In many ways it was similar to that of the letter referred to above. As in all of CAE's work, the artists were investigating a chain of decisions highly relevant to the public, but from which the public had been largely excluded.

In the United States since 2000, there has been a six-fold increase in annual spending for biodefense. A lot of this money is going toward the construction of several new biosafety level 4 labs in different parts of the country. Because these facilities are built for research into deadly infectious pathogens, they are capital-intensive complexes with high-tech security systems that have to be maintained around the clock. All the people working in these labs from the scientists to the janitors have to be restricted, their backgrounds checked and their daily routines subject to intense surveillance. In addition, the major public funding opportunities for research in universities are becoming severely skewed towards biodefense so that labs in educational institutions will also be subject to high security restrictions, affecting the culture of the entire institution, making it more hostile to the free and open sharing of research materials and information.

CAE's work would point out that the threat of bioterrorism is actually very unlikely because, from a weapons point of view, with the exception of anthrax,[15] biological agents are unstable, hard to work with, and a lot more trouble than explosives and chemical toxins. We should also know that the problem with an aggressive biodefense program is that it is essentially indistinguishable from an aggressive bioweapons program; that the new biosafety level 4 labs will actually be developing new deadly pathogens in order to figure out how to defend against them and that these facilities may actually increase the likelihood of previously unknown lethal microbes; that in the only bioterrorism scare in the United States, the anthrax anonymously sent through the mail was traced back to one of the government defense labs studying bioweapons, and three years after that discovery the government still can't locate the perpetrator.[16] And as concerns the signatories to the letter cited above, increased biodefense spending comes at the expense of research into common infectious diseases that kill millions of people every year. What if we started thinking about the militarization of public health and the corporatization of all things military? What if we looked at who is gaining from contracts to build and maintain these high security facilities?

Most scientists who criticize the Bush administration's science policy are taken off committees, have their recommendations rewritten, are denied access to policy boards and funding, or are just ignored.[17] Scientists who criticize the direction favored by corporate science risk losing funding or having their careers ruined.

In CAE's case the FBI stumbled onto the materials of a group of artists preparing a very thorough and knowledgeable critique of policy that relates to capital, science, politics, terrorism, and the mother of all four, the military techno-security cineplex. But couldn't they see that what they found was art?

Legibility And Legality

Sometime last year I saw a picture of Boston College student Joseph Previtera staging a protest outside a U.S. Armed Forces Recruiting Office. The image's effect was immediate because Previtera had donned a sack-like shift that came to his knees and a pointed cloth hood that covered his face and head. He stood on a crate with arms outstretched and dangled a couple of stereo wires, thus silently impersonating the tortured prisoner of Abu Ghraib for over an hour before the Boston police arrested him for disturbing the peace. By the time he got to the station the charges were two felonies: false report of the location of explosives and a hoax device. In other words, the wires coming from his sleeves clearly indicated a false bomb threat. Fortunately these charges did not hold up to an indictment.

For a split second I joked to myself, "The government needs to go to art school. Don't they get it?"

But of course they get it. They get it all too well. "They" understand that an expressive means, in this case performance, is being engaged to make a statement critical of U.S. policy and actions abroad. They refuse to recognize there is a difference between the use of an expressive means to make a critical statement and the use of a substance or technology to pose a threat. This illiteracy is not simply a matter of ignorance or a misunderstanding that can be cleared up after an earnest discussion. This is a willful dysfunction that is serving the government, not only in ratcheting up the number of terror-related suspects it can report busting, but in clearing the public sphere of ungovernable reality.

If the developing legal framework defines terrorism and its support as any thought or expression that might undermine the U.S. government and the transnational capitalist functionaries it fronts, even if only by dissenting from it, art as a category is not protected. Ideas, expression, and communication, as categories, are not protected. Artists, academics, intellectuals, activists, clergy, anyone–hopefully everyone–who lives the premise that they are free to openly speak their beliefs and pursue their questions has reason to take this issue as their own.

One reason the First Amendment becomes moot in the current legal cosmos is that the realm of the symbolic is not recognized as distinct. For the Bush administration ideology is reality. Just as "reality-based" science, or evidence against weapons of mass destruction, or realistic assessments of a war in Iraq are not recognized as phenomena with imposing significance, symbolic adversaries may be prosecuted to the full extent of the law–and to the full extent that the law can be distorted and mangled.

A series of very unfortunate events bestowed on the FBI a reason to investigate Steve Kurtz. They found material critical of corporate capital and its uses of science, and, where relevant, of U.S. policy. Like most politically motivated people, for Kurtz the point of producing such material was to publish it; the FBI could have found the same material in many places had they been looking, because its legality is a cornerstone of our society. We don't know if CAE was already being monitored, but circumstances put them under the government's scrutiny as could happen to any of us. Given the excuse and the complete authority to investigate every aspect of Kurtz's life, the U.S. Justice Department found a minor, noncriminal irregularity on which, as has become the form, they pinned criminal charges. It is not conspiratorial to say that the charges also serve the right wing agenda, including the maintenance and enforcement of divisions of knowledge and ever-harsher penalties for intellectual property violations, because these things become endemic to a system. The prosecution does not have to articulate the goals of the system even to itself; everything is already in place.

Of course it's about the art. It's about representation. The individual cases, the kinds of cases, the facts of the cases, the arguments related to the cases, the numbers of cases and the distortions of those numbers, these too are very much matters of representation. The case against the Palestinians, the case against Islam, the case against pacifists, the case against independent science, the case against rural people who don't conceive of their knowledge as property, the case against all people who are in the way of the cannibalistic machine of global capital cannot only be won by force. It has to be fought in the field of representation, because we know too much. And because our legal system and ideals actually provide vigorous correctives to abuses of power—but only if we fight for them. What is clear is that those correctives, the right to free speech, to open and collective knowledge, to equality of race and religion, and to accountability and transparency of power, have to be actively reclaimed as a matter of daily life.

And they have to be reclaimed in every arena where proto-fascism infests governance: in the police and the courts, in the establishment of racialized hierarchies, in ethnic and financial exclusions from education, in the restriction of creative endeavor, in the criminalization of curiosity, and in the monoculture of private property as the single medium of meaningful human exchange.

[1] The opinions in this paper are those of the author and not necessarily of the CAE Defense Fund. However, I would like to acknowledge the invaluable collective input of all of the defense team in developing these analyses.

[2] *Department of Justice Data Manual.*

[3] Cole, David, "Taking Liberties," *The Nation*, October 4, 2004.

[4] Gourevitch, Alexander, "Body Count, How John Ashcroft's Inflated Terrorism Statistics Undermine the War on Terrorism," *The Washington Monthly*, June 2003.

[5] *Criminal Terrorism Enforcement Since the 9/11/01 Attacks, A TRAC Special Report*, December 8, 2003.

[6] See Jane Meyer's "Outsourcing Torture," *The New Yorker*, Issue February 14, 2005, http://www.newyorker.com/fact/content/?050214fa_fact6.

[7] Both Richard Reid and Jose Padilla tried to be part of al Qaeda, but true to its notorious insularity, the network gave

these foreign converts a generic training and sent them back to the west. It was Padilla's idea to make a dirty bomb, but they never gave him a plan.

[8] In December 2005, Sami al-Arian was acquitted on 7 of 15 charges. On the remaining 8 charges the jury was deadlocked. The future of this case is still uncertain.

[9] Brandon Mayfield is suing the U.S. government for violating his rights and also contending that the USA PATRIOT Act is unconstitutional. His attorneys have requested the Justice Department disclose exactly what secret searches were made in the investigation and have received a letter acknowledging that the PATRIOT Act was used. This may be the first time a citizen has secured such information about the PATRIOT Act.

[10] Sami Omar Al-Hussayen, a Saudi Ph.D. candidate in computer science, was acquitted by an Idaho jury in June 2004 of terrorism charges for setting up and running websites that prosecutors said were used to recruit terrorists, raise money, and disseminate inflammatory rhetoric. The jury deadlocked on other counts of visa fraud and false statements. These nonterrorism charges were dropped when Al-Hussayen and his family agreed to deportation.

[11] Marcus Garvey was convicted of mail fraud relating to the finances of the failed Black Star (shipping) Line. By most accounts, his enemies were not just the government, but prominent black businessmen who had decided his cause was not in their interests. He served one year in the Atlanta penitentiary and was then deported to Jamaica.

[12] US DOJ, *United States Attorneys Manual, Title 9, Criminal*

Resource Manual, http://www.usdoj.gov/usao/eousa/foia_reading_room/usam/title9/43mcrm.htm.

[13] On January 13, 2005, the Center for Food Safety published a comprehensive report on Monsanto's lawsuits and threats against farmers. The 84-page report is available at http://www.centerforfoodsafety.org/Monsantovsusfarmersreport.cfm.

[14] Please see http://www.ucsusa.org/scientific_integrity.

[15] While the organism itself can be stabilized in spore form, it is still very difficult to work with. Normally it lives in the ground at a very low density. To increase density to a military grade (of around a billion spores per gram) and keep it moving through the air is difficult. Moreover, the natural instability of weather conditions make it impossible to predict how it will move once released. Of the two field releases–October 2001 in the United States and in Russia in 1979–casualty rates were exceptionally low, certainly not even close to WMD potential.

[16] For examples, see Judith Miller, "New Germ Labs Stir a Debate over Secrecy and Safety," *The New York Times*, February 10, 2004; Dan Vergano and Steve Sternberg, "Anthrax Slip-Ups Raise Fears about Planned Biolabs," *USA Today*, October 13, 2004; and "What Exactly Is the Army Up To?" *Deseret Morning News*, July 25, 2004; and especially Rick Weiss and Susan Schmidt, "Capitol Hill Anthrax Matches Army's Stocks," *The Washington Post*, December 6, 2001.

[17] Please see the Restoring Scientific Integrity website for specific examples at http://www.ucsusa.org.

Critical Art Ensemble's books address the deep-rooted replication of capitalism at the frontiers of science and technology. Whether discussing robotics, information technologies, or the biological sciences, CAE skillfully exposes the hidden agendas at the foundation of 21st-century life, and suggest interventions and semiotic shocks that could collectively negate the rising intensity of authoritarian culture.

All books available from Autonomedia <www.autonomedia.org>

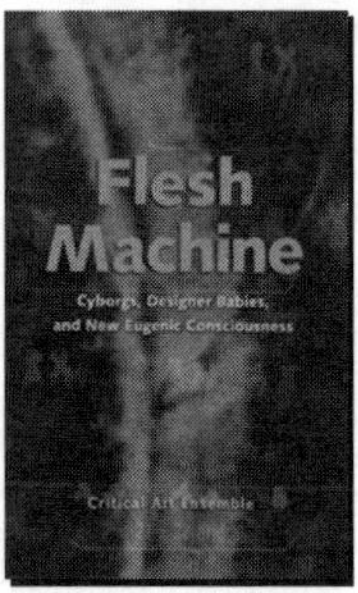

In **Flesh Machine: Cyborgs, Designer Babies, and the New Eugenic Consciousness**, Critical Art Ensemble focuses its sights on the new frontier of pan-capital – the political and economic development of flesh products and services. CAE begins mapping this development in *Flesh Machine* by examining the use of reproductive technologies to achieve an intensified degree of control over worker and consumer-citizen. This book aims to establish a counter-narrative to the spectacular promises of the life industries.

1998 156 pp 4.5" x 7" $9.95

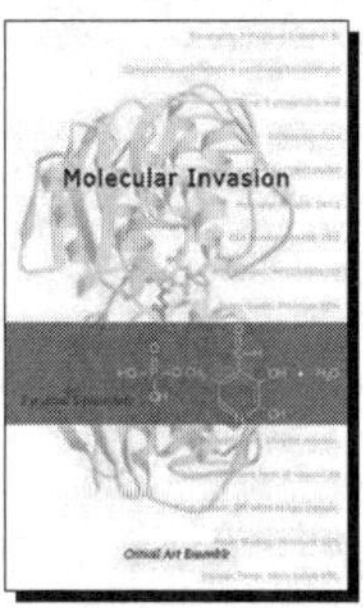

Molecular Invasion acts as a companion to *Flesh Machine*, articulating the politics of transgenics, developing a model for the creation of a contestational biology, and providing direct interventionist tactics intended to disrupt this assault on the organic realm. Includes the essays "Fuzzy Biological Sabotage" and "Transgenic Production and Cultural Resistance: A Seven-Point Plan."

2002 140 pp 4.5" x 7" $9.95

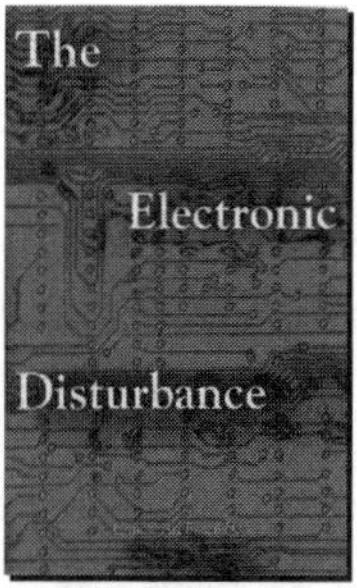

The Electronic Disturbance is the first collection of essays and short pieces explaining the nature of nomadic power and resistance in the age of the virtual. "The current technological revolution has created a new geography of power relations—as data, human beings confront an authoritarial impulse that thrives on absence. As a virtual geography of cognizance and action, resistance must assert itself in electronic space."

1994 | 156 pp | 4.5" x 7" | $9.95

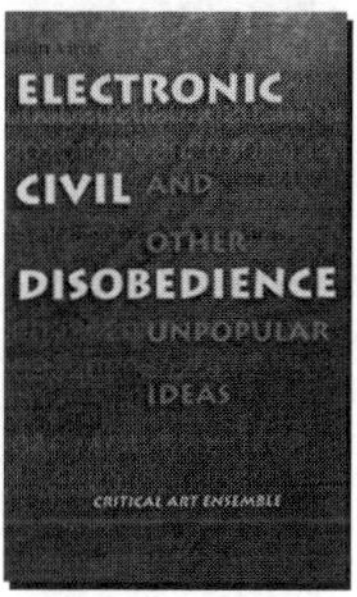

Electronic Civil Disobedience continues where *The Electronic Disturbance* leaves off, suggesting strategies of resistance to nomadic power, and investigating tactics of nonrationality to get at the core of autonomy. Fusing a situationist-influenced concept of contestational art, an understanding of the parallel nature of cultural and political action borrowed from Gramsci, and a hacker's understanding of how new technology functions, *Electronic Civil Disobedience* refines an understanding of the nature of power and resistance in the information age.

1996 | 144 pp | 4.5" x 7" | $9.95

Digital Resistance: Explorations in Tactical Media completes a tryptych on the theory and practice of nomadic opposition to Power. Beginning with a discussion of "tactical media" as a mode of creative opposition outside of traditional political activism, the book presents eight essays illustrating the breadth of opportunities tactical media makes possible.

2001 | 192 pp | 6" x 9" | $14.00

New Autonomy

a series of books from Autonomedia tracing the border between politics and culture, the New Left and the Newer Left, the academy and the street.

Jim Fleming & Peter Lamborn Wilson, Editors

TAZ: The Temporary Autonomous Zone, Ontological Anarchy, Poetic Terrorism
Hakim Bey

This Is Your Final Warning!
Thom Metzger

Friendly Fire
Bob Black

The Lizard Club
Steve Abbott

First and Last Emperors
Kenneth Dean & Brian Massumi

This World We Must Leave and Other Essays
Jacques Camatte

Future Primitive
John Zerzan

Whore Carnival
Shannon Bell

Invisible Governance: Essays in African Micropolitics
David Hecht & Maliqalim Simone

X Texts
Derek Pell

Pirate Utopias: Moorish Corsairs and European Renegadoes
Peter Lamborn Wilson

The Electronic Disturbance
Electronic Civil Disobedience
Digital Resistance
Flesh Machine
Molecular Invasion
Marching Plague
Critical Art Ensemble

Unholy Bible: Hebrew Literature of the Kingdom Period
Jacob Rabinowitz

The Root Is Man
Dwight MacDonald

The Devil's Anarchy
Stephan Snelders

Between Dog and Wolf: Essays on Art and Politics
David Levi Strauss

Social Overload
Pierre-Henri Jeudy

Caliban and the Witch
Silvia Federici

bolo'bolo
p.m.

Free Cooperation
Christoph Spehr

Unleashing the Collective Phantoms
Brian Holmes
